I'm Grrreat!

One Man's Choice to Live Joyfully

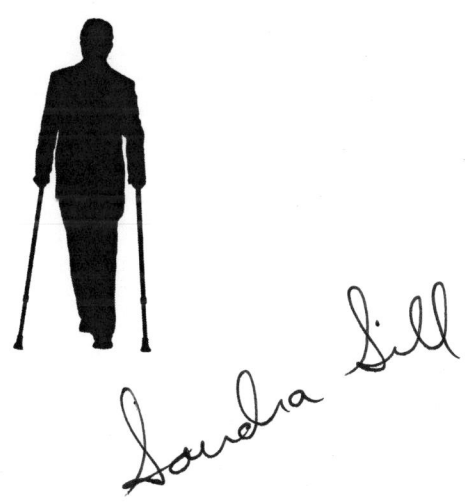

Edward & Sandra Sill

Copyright © 2012 by Sandra Sill

All rights reserved. Published by Aperture Press. Name and associated logos are trademarks and/or registered trademarks of Aperture Press, LLC.

No part of this publication may be reproduced, stored in a retrieval system, or transmitted in any form or by any means, electronic, mechanical, photocopying, recording, or otherwise, without written permission of the publisher. For information, write to Aperture Press, P.O. Box 6485, Reading, PA 19610 or visit www.AperturePress.net.

ISBN 978-0-9850026-5-7
Library of Congress Control Number: 2012940205

Printed in the U.S.A.

First Edition, June 2012

Edited by Dick Conklin
Cover & interior design by Stephen Wagner

*This book is dedicated to the medical profession,
hospitals, medical colleges, drug companies, nurses,
doctors, caregivers, and my wife, Sandie.*
—*Ed Sill*

Also our children, friends, and neighbors.
—*Sandra Sill*

Contents

Introduction 7

The Early Years 11

Back to High School 35

Sandie Meets Ed 47

More Bad News 69

Some Funny Stuff 95

In Their Own Words 111

Introduction

My husband Ed Sill started writing a book about himself because family and friends were pushing him to do it. We knew he was failing, and probably about the time he had the last cancer scare around 2004, he finally started writing some things down. His writing hand was not working well, and he felt numbness and tingling. We at first thought it must be the chemo and radiation treatments that caused it. Ed said that maybe it was carpal tunnel syndrome, and went to see a doctor who operated on it. Now we realize that it probably was not carpal tunnel but polio syndrome. He stopped writing the book and my daughters and I suggested that he use a tape recorder; this is all that Ed left us on the tape recorder.

He went into a downhill spiral in August of 2005. He passed away on January 10, 2006 with a diagnosis of poliomyelitis.

In this book, Ed talks about boyhood adventures, family vacations, neighborhoods, schools, friends, politics, meeting me, Sandie, living with polio, and his multiple battles with cancer.

I have tried to finish his story but I know that my explanations may not be as colorful as the way he might explain things. People who knew him knew that he had quite a way with words and could stretch things "just a little."

–Sandie

What This Book's Title Means

Since Ed was dealing with polio in his teens and cancer since he was 40, he was always being asked how he was feeling.

His response was usually, "I'm Grrreat!" or" Terrrific!" or "Fannntastic"

I felt that needed to be in the title to show his attitude toward the challenges he had in his lifetime. This is a man who could have been defined by these challenges but never focused on them.

He focused on living.

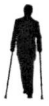

The Early Years

On October 5, 1940, I was born to Francis and Irene Sill. Life for me started at Brady Maternity Hospital in Albany, New York. The other member of the household was a sister named Irene. Later on, 15 years later, the parents were to surprise the family with two more blessings. I helped to select the name of the new additions, the boy was named Frances Charles and at the time he seemed light as a "feather", which became his nickname. A girl born around two years later was named Patricia Irene. My parents' life was a series of struggles and trials like most families go through. My father's job was a brakeman for the New York Central Railroad and my mother was a hairdresser.

In the early years, like many young married couples, my parents moved quite frequently. We started on Broad Street in the south end of the City of Albany. Some of our relatives lived in the same proximity, being mostly of Irish, German and Roman Catholic beliefs.

Hawk Street was our next stop, across from the Hanlon family; they were in the ash and trash hauling business, successful, wonderful folks, with a son, Jim, who became my friend. One early recollection made an impression on me; my Uncle Ken, acting as a Civil Defense leader, had to make sure lights were out at night and window shades down. It was feared enemy planes could spot lights to help bomb an area. During WW II, every precaution was taken to aid the civilians.

Our next move was to 169 Third Avenue. Fond memories abounded there, as the Moran family was our neighbors. Dick Moran was my age; we dared each other to enter the Gotchaw brickyard, where many boyhood dreams began. We caught garden snakes, frogs, tadpoles, lightning bugs and butterflies. Many species took refuge there. Kid treasures for sure, but also a source of teenage and adult entertainment as well. The place was loaded with old lumber and bricks. We built forts for our pretend gunfights; the bricks served that purpose fine.

Election Day Fires

In the fall, wood was salvaged for Election Day fires, a tradition to celebrate a custom of the time: welcoming new politicians into office. People of all ages would come to the yard and load wood on old horse-drawn wagons. They brought the wood to empty fields and made a bonfire. They placed tires around fire hydrants, to delay putting the fires out. The flames would get so hot and high that telephone lines and electric cables would melt and sometimes windows would break. The Fire Department was kept busy all night going from field to field to control the blazes. This custom continued for many years.

Winter always brought fun, hauling our sleighs, skis, toboggans and plastic sheets up the slopes toward Second Avenue. The first hill was easy to climb but not the second one. The ride down was worth all the risks and dangers, if you could stay on the trail. A path worn on the hill threw you where it wanted, so you sometimes went over the side into brush and trees and would come home with cuts or bruises. We also used the First Avenue alley ending up near Elizabeth Street, a mile away. The chance of accidents was very high as delivery trucks for milk or coal were always around this street. On one occasion, I found myself under a coal truck bleeding profusely from my head. So between Gotshaw's brickyard in the summer and winter sports on the slopes, there was always mischief to get into. Baseball filled in our dull times as you could always round up kids for a game of baseball or basketball.

My parents bought a home at 93 Clinton Avenue around 1945. We lived in a four-story apartment house in the bottom floor. The top three floors had beautiful mirrors, very ornate and about eight feet tall and four feet wide. The Fisher family lived on the second floor and were the first to have a TV; they invited all the tenants to come and see Kukla, Fran and Ollie, Milton Berle's Texaco Hour, Your Show of Shows with Sid Caesar and Imogene Coco, Superman, Amos and Andy, the Lone Ranger, and Hopalong Cassidy were—all popular shows at the time. My best pal lived a block down the street next to the Garland Funeral Home. One day we were having one of our snowball fights and broke a window at Garland's. We were pretty scared but the Garlands turned out to be very understanding about how young kids could get into mischief and break windows, especially with a snowball. So they were very fair and only asked our parents to pay for the window.

We rode our bikes to school at *Philip Livingston Junior High* after leaving Public School #4. We all felt like big shots and kept them locked in the school cellar. The Principal was Charlie Walker, a real tough man. One time he was attacked by some teens with a knife; he handled that situation and came out on top. There were other similar rumors about how he always prevailed. He was like a hero to local folks.

Rensselaerville, Lake Myosotis, and the Huyck Preserve

I was about 8 years old and my sister 11, when my dad built a small two-bedroom camp on land owned by the Huyck Preserve at Lake Myosotis. As many other summer people did, we rented the land from the preserve that we later learned was owned by a company in Rensselaer. We spent about four summers there, catching fish, exploring waterfalls, catching tadpoles and frogs, rowing boats and swimming. We ventured there in early spring one year. Snow was still melting and ice was visible on the lake. The icy dock was very slippery and can you guess who slipped on it and wound up in the lake? There I went, down to the bottom, counting bubbles as they passed. Luckily, my sister saw my plight and grabbed me by my snowsuit collar. She held me alongside of the dock, hollering for help until the caretaker, Alan Davis, ran down to pull me out—cold and soaking wet. I was about 10 pounds heavier, maybe more. That was a scary experience, one lesson you can never forget.

While we camped at Lake Myosotis, one summer my Dad and Mom became acquainted with Dr. Thomas Ordway and his wife, Jenny. The doctor was very well known at Albany Medical Center hospital, a teaching professor at the medical college and a doctor at the hospital. The doctor's family lived in the Albany Shaker Road area, a well-kept, well-to-do area near Latham. Their summer home was about a mile or two from our campsite. We were invited to his old colonial farmhouse many times after our parents and the Ordways became good friends. My dad did some chauffeuring for the doctor, as he was getting on in age. We were invited to their summer house to ride horses. There were several horses, a couple of barns, a carriage shed and several other structures on the land. He had a caretaker for the farm when he couldn't be there and there was some question as to whether the animals were being taken care of the way they should have been. The custodial people sometimes were accused of not seeing to their needs, like getting water to them on time, or not grooming them, or riding them. One horse was a big black Morgan named Beau; he was about 16 hands high and as a young lad of 12, he stood and towered over me like a big statue. I was allowed to ride him and he usually had one thing on his mind, to take you up into an orchard, brush you off on a tree and run back to the barn and start eating grain. My sister Rena rode a big jumper; she jumped over structures on the farm and got along well with the horse, building a relationship and going to horse shows. My sister won several ribbons working with the jumper. They became quite a team.

That was a fun summer. We learned a lot on the 100-acre farm. It had beautiful pine trees that were planted early in the doctor's career. They were set in rows, reminding you of church pews that were so precise you would look through them like you were looking into a time tunnel. You could see animals playing, squirrels, chipmunks, sometimes ermine, and lots of wildlife. It was quite a wild refuge actually, with that much land it only stood that in the early fifties you would see plenty of wildlife and we did.

I have a friend who always tells me, "You have to go back, you have to go back in time to tell the history of events that are going to happen in the future, or history repeats itself." His name was Don Brady, and he was very influential in part of my life when we were involved in sports, in managing Little League, Senior Babe Ruth League and Babe Ruth League teams in Rensselaer. So we will go back, once again—I want to take you back to some of the impressionable things that happened while we were camping at Lake Myosotis.

One year we helped the New York State Conservation Department net and tag fish for a study on their growth habits and several other conditions that the state was interested in, to see how much the fish not only grew, but what their eating habits were, where they migrated to feed on other wildlife, and what areas of the lake were best suited for different types of fish. It was fun, and we learned quite a bit that we hadn't known about nature.

One of the most enjoyable times was the leisure time listening to old radio shows. I tried not to miss The Shadow Knows, The Green Hornet, Von Monroe, The Lux Video Theater, and many detective shows like Dick Tracy. Singers Perry Como and Dinah Shore were popular at the time and we loved listening to their shows.

After the camp was torn down and re-assembled as a year-round home, we decided to live there permanently, moving from 93 Clinton Avenue in Albany. The foundation needed to be dug out and it was decided that I would do most of that work. I used a shovel and a wheelbarrow and would take it down a series of planks to a large sand pit and dump the dirt in that sand pit. It took a whole summer to finish and the only good part was that it was a powdered composition that was not real heavy, unless it was wet. Usually you would have to dig several feet before the sand became real wet.

My father didn't like not being able to own the campsite land and then the Preserve started to raise our rent each year. He decided to tear down the camp and rebuild it on land he had purchased on Church Road, off Western Avenue in the town of Westmere, some 28 miles from the site that the camp was presently standing on. Boy, did I get a real firsthand view of what hard work was really like! Back then, as a 12-year-old lad, I learned how to accomplish many things.

The next project was to build a road that would, more or less, circle the house. This driveway was built with multiple compositions. It started with a layer of rock, ashes and cinders over the rock, a layer of blacktop a couple of inches over that, and finally there was about 6 to 8 inches of concrete over the roadbed. We then took boards and shimmied them back and forth to make ridges in the cement so in the winter you could get better traction on the cement. We were successful, which took quite a bit of time, but it turned out really well.

New Home, New School

I first attended Guilderland Junior-Senior High School in 1954, which was a new adventure for me. Since the school was some 20 miles from my home, I had to ride a school bus. The school was very new, big, and roomy with large fields for athletic activities, and the gym was used for various events with the stands folding up into the walls. A friend of mine, Joan Milne from Philip Livingston Junior High had also moved to Westmere in my school district. We had been in the same classes and wound up friends for some 46 years. We still saw each other at class reunions, like at our 45th where we got to see most of our old chums, except for the thirteen who had passed away. *(Joan passed away in March 2006, two months after Ed.)*

One of these school pals was Arnold Stalker. He was a class clown and was always coming up with gimmicks to make everyone laugh. At times he would use a rubber band with a washer and put it in book and would lift up his rear end gently, a little at a time. Soon the washer would spin and make it sound like he was breaking wind. He seemed to do this the most in Mr. Sharkey's English class, which was kind of boring so he would try to liven things up. He was always trying to protect the meek and mild kids from the big bullies. He had many fisticuffs bouts with these bullies and always either held his own or came out on top. He was sent home several times and suspended quite a few days during the year. (*Arnie passed away in 1997).*

Our school was classified as a B School, so we competed in the Central Hudson Valley League with rivals Colonie, Bethlehem, Shenendehowa and many other schools. Baseball was my best sport. We had a super coach named Fred Field and I also played JV and freshman ball under the JV coach, Mike Kopcza. My catchers were Dick Brunk and Bob Gould.

During one game I pitched against Albany Academy I didn't have a full uniform. The other team laughed and taunted me for the way I looked. It was probably a mistake on their part, because after taunting me for 9 innings we won the game 9 to 1.

The funny part of the game was Coach Kopcza, who kept telling me he was going to teach me how to throw a curve ball.

He would watch me pitch in warm-ups and I naturally didn't try to throw many breaking balls because it was early in the season and you could hurt your elbow. Well, he changed his mind after he saw that I already had quite a curve ball and I was breaking off in another game pretty well and the curve was not only curving but it was dropping.

I went on to win four games in my freshman year. The coach said it looked like I was going to be a great prospect for my next three years of high school. In the fall, I went out for the football team. It was hard work as I had chores to do at home and with my school work and homework, it was hard to keep on top of everything. Well, as you might guess, I got hurt, spraining my left leg and knee. The boys in the neighborhood would still try to get me to play baseball, basketball, and whatever. Well, instead of trying to rest, I went and tried to make the difference of having a team or not having a team.

(*An article in Ed's high school newspaper dated Friday, November 12, 1954 was titled, "Music Groups Featured in School Assembly." It described a November 5th program at the Guilderland Central High School featuring the first appearance of the "Harmonizers," a new Junior High School boys' chorus. The article listed the songs they were singing and the names of boys who were singing in the first, second and third parts. Edward Sill was in the third part.*

A 1956 article on the school newspaper sports page, "Guilderland Central Track Meet Held April 27," reported Ed as placing third in the Junior High 100-yard Dash.

Ed told us that he became ill one night with chills and fever. His father was digging a basement under their home and he had to do a lot of the digging and hauling of the dirt. That was something he did the day before he became ill, along with playing football and being exhausted.
—Sandie)

Bad News: A Diagnosis of Polio

Around October of 1956 I came down with polio, one of the two last people in the area to come down with this disease. Terry Cohom was the other person; she and I spent days in the hospital together. I was jealous of Terry because she could do things that I couldn't do, like jumping up on the table for her exams. They wanted to find out how much damage was done to her muscles as well as me. *(Ed had never received the polio vaccine. His family was told to get vaccinated right away.)*

My story was, like my old friend said, "you have to go back." Our family doctor was Dr. Bohlan. He came out when my mom called him and said that I seemed to have some kind of flu type condition. He examined me and wasn't sure what I had, so he treated me for a flu bug. My illness did not go away and I soon got much sicker than I had been. The second time he came he recognized that there was a big problem, so he called an ambulance and I was rushed off to the *Albany Medical Center*.

He diagnosed it as polio and it looked like this was going to be a real big change in my life and I was pretty scared, to say the least. I was put in a quarantined or contagious area. An iron lung was wheeled in to my bedside. Luckily, I did not have to go in it but I lost 30 pounds the first week I was in the hospital. I had to be catheterized, for my own protection, as I had trouble going to the bathroom and had to have sand bags on each side of my legs to make sure that after the disease runs its course the legs and feet do not get what they call "drop foot." You can be deformed by this disease and it can do quite a bit of damage to your muscles and movement.

The doctor for my rehabilitation was Dr. Thomas Gormley; he was a polio specialist and the boss of the physical therapy department. The staff at AMC did what they could to help. They really didn't deal with rehab long term. They would put you in a Hubbard water tank to relax your muscles and move or warm your body. They would do some stretching of the muscles so your legs would move freely the way they were supposed to move but it was not for long term care.

During the time that I was an outpatient at Albany Medical Center hospital, the *March of Dimes* came in to aid my rehabilitation. I had a personal driver who would pick me up two or three times a week; her name was Ann Trager. She was a wonderful person who would drive me to and from my exercise classes and rehab at Albany Med and she would deliver other patients and pick up people on a schedule. She was always running during the day for any of the disabled people in different areas that her organization was helping out. They would work with the doctors and nurses and try to do everything they could do to help with their rehabilitation. It was a wonderful, wonderful organization.

From Albany Medical Center to Sunnyview Rehab Hospital

Next, I was sent to Sunnyview Rehab Hospital in Schenectady, which was a specialized rehabilitation center. It was quite a hospital, as you could not only get your treatments every day but you could also attend school right on site. They would wheel your bed right down to the classroom or you could roll yourself down to the class, if you were physically able to use a wheelchair. I made a lot of friends and felt I didn't have to lose a lot of time from regular school classes while I was rehabilitating, and hopefully I would be able to pick up where I left off when I got sick. The teacher, Ms. Wolfe, had quite a personality and was extremely school-oriented and wanted to make sure that her teaching became as much a part of my life as the rehabilitation.

Every Saturday night we watched wrestling. Lights were out by 9 o'clock for certain age groups. One guy in our room didn't have to have lights out until 11 o'clock. Wrestling started at 11 o'clock.

I was in a room with three other guys. Mike McCusker was from Keysville; he had polio and his fingers were cramped up so they looked like arthritis. Other than that, he had one leg brace and could get around fairly well.

The second boy in the room was Paul Stacey. I learned that he had lived in the south end of Albany where I did, down around the Broad Street, First Avenue Alley and Hawk Street area. He was quite an interesting case. He was driving a compression tractor in the Catskills during hay time. The motor on the tractor went off and he had no brakes so he panicked. It started down the hill and hit a huge stone. He fell off the tractor and was run over by the rear wheel, almost severing his spine. He was in a hammock and they would flip him over every four hours, so he would lie on his back for four hours and on his front for four hours. Needless to say, it was not a very comfortable position for that kid no matter what happened.

The third guy in the room, Tony, had escaped from a reform school. He was only about 16 at the time and he had traveled around looking for food. According to him, he went into a barn near a farmhouse and must have made some noise because the farmer came out and shot him with a shotgun. He was now a paraplegic, with no use of his legs, no feeling from the waist down and his legs would jump from muscle spasms. He was in a wheelchair. It was quite a sad story. It made you appreciate your family and what you had in life when you wound up as a roommate with people in this category.

The funny part was watching wrestling every Saturday night. We had a nurse that we use to call "Old Combat Boots" and it was her task to come around between 11 and 12 and make sure everyone was honoring the lights-off policy. What we would do, when Mike had to go to bed at 11, he would shut off the last remaining light over his bed and shut the TV off. As soon as Combat Boots came around and made her bed check we would sneak the TV back on, make sure the door was closed and keep the volume low and try to watch wrestling until midnight. Well, as you might know, a couple of times she snuck up on us, caught us and there was heck to pay. We learned how to be quieter when we did it; I think we wound up using a towel or blanket over the TV so we could reflect the light in a certain way so she would leave us alone. It worked but we did get caught.

One of the other funny recollections I have of Sunnyview, which was a most pleasant time in some ways, was my physical therapist, Connie. She had jet black hair, blue Irish eyes and she was just a very, very pretty girl. She was, at the time, about 22 years old, an Irish lass with certainly strong feelings toward Ireland. She was very, very concerned with what was going on at that time, problems between the Irish Republican Army (IRA) and England. It almost made one feel that she did support their efforts to oust the English or overthrow them from governing their country. I always had the feeling that she may have donated to help the rebels buy arms or do things of that nature. A lot of people in Ireland did not like the English running their country and supervising everything they did. After three months of tumbling with her on mats, in and out the pool and stretching exercises and working out with her constantly, it became almost more than a companion thing. I was very young at the time, and I certainly didn't know much about love matters, except puppy love.

On one occasion, after I was able to get into a wheelchair and ride around the halls, we were going to a social event. For some reason, someone teased Connie, my physical therapist, into riding on my lap. Well, as you might know, a doctor caught her and told her it was very unprofessional to be riding on a patient's lap and certainly did not have a good appearance for other hospital patients. She certainly caught heck for that one and I think that there was more than just a patient attraction on her part to me.

Later on in life, after I got out of the hospital, she came to visit me several times. And there again, I was certainly too young to know the ways of love, so I really didn't understand why she kept coming to see me. But I can tell you that they were more than just social visits as several times from the conversation it lead me to believe that she really missed me and that it was more than just a teacher/patient relationship. It wound up ending there, as it was certainly no place I was going to go with it at the time, being a younger person.

One of the highlights of being at Sunnyview, was when a professional boxer came to visit us and he gave everybody a little pair of boxing gloves with his name on it: Carmen Basillio. He was a lightweight champion or contender at the time. Other celebrities came to the hospital at times to visit the patients and cheer us up. Other good times were the Christmas shows when they would put on a show and give all the kids and adult patients' presents donated by Schenectady area businesses. So there were a lot of fond memories that came out of Sunnyview, and although I have never gotten a chance to go back there and visit, I certainly should take the time to see how much it's changed. I have heard it has become bigger and more important in the Capital District than when I was there.

Mike McCusker, in our room, who was about 19 at the time, fell in love with one of the other patients, Judy Allen. She was about 16 and from the Scotia area. It was fun to watch, and it may have been puppy love. They would go around on their wheelchairs together. They would go to class and movies and almost everything together. Wherever you saw Judy, you saw Mike; they were inseparable. I tried to find Mike several years later in the Keysville area. I was unable to find his house up there; just out of curiosity I wanted to find out whether he and Judy had gotten married, as it seemed like more than puppy love at the time.

I spent about four months in rehabilitation at Sunnyview. I was quite concerned that my schooling was getting in the way of my physical therapy. There were times that the teacher, Mrs. Cusperd, actually would come to my mat classes or swimming classes or stretching out exercises and try to take me from that activity and bring me back to the school class. I was quite perturbed at the time as I felt that my health and well being and physical condition were more important than schooling. After several of these episodes of being taken out of my physical therapy classes, I approached my mother with it during visiting hours several times and after awhile she was quite concerned herself and was not too happy to hear my complaints about having to go to school classes instead of physical therapy classes. She asked me what I would like to do about it and I said at this point I would like to quit school and go back to Guilderland Central High School after my rehab was more complete and we knew where I was going to stand and how I was going to move about.

Hopefully, when you are in a rehab hospital you plan to come out in pretty good shape. In my case, I was quite a sight. I wound up having to wear double leg braces as my muscles were very weak in both legs and I also had to wear what they call a hook corset around my waist because my stomach muscles were also hit pretty bad. As a matter of fact, at Albany Medical Center I was lucky to lift my arms and feed myself. I was very weak and this disease is one that can really destabilize anybody. As I improved and got my double leg braces, I was trained how to go up and down stairs and fall, as you can certainly hurt yourself when you trip over something or got clumsy and wound up falling on the ground or an object. You had to reinvent the wheel and learn how to handle yourself all over again.

Back Home Again

I was up on my leg braces for one week when I asked my mother to have Dr. Gormley sign me out of the hospital and allow me to come home where I would do my own rehabilitation program and try to get myself back on my feet before the new school year started.

My classmates used to come up during visiting hours, usually about 7 to 9 pm on weeknights. They were pretty nice and bought me a portable TV, so I could have a TV in my bedroom when I went home. They wanted to do something nice for me and I was pretty popular in my freshman class. A lot of classmates felt pretty bad that I was one of the last people to get polio in the Tri-City area, so it was especially gratifying to know that they would take up a collection and do what they could to get me something nice. I really appreciated that and it made you feel that you wanted to get into rehabilitation and back into the mainstream and dealing with your friends and going to school.

It was quite a trying time; I have a recollection of coming home and learned that walking with two leg braces was not an easy task. I also had to use Canadian crutches and several times when I was walking around the yard I would trip over the tree roots and wound up either knocking myself out when my head hit a tree or come down on the ground pretty hard, winding up with several bruises. I soon learned I really had to walk on level land. I had a 1949 Nash Rambler at my disposal that my father had given me as a present for when I could drive. So I had older boys drive me up and down our hilly driveway, which was like the side of a mountain, then I would be on the level of Church Road and started out walking to the corner of Church and Zorn Road, which was a very short distance.

I would do this several times a week and gradually try to increase my distance and get more and more exercise to the point that I was able to throw one of my leg braces away. Then I would only have to deal with the other one and the hook corset, which I was able to accomplish in a few short months. However, the bigger problem was my left leg—the muscles had deteriorated to the size and strength of a six year old carrying the weight of a fifteen year old. It wasn't a very comfortable situation. I tried to do sit-ups and work out on the mats just like I did in the hospital and I gradually was able to get rid of the hooked corset. Then I was able to do more and more because it kind of blocked a lot of the exercises and things that your stomach muscles could perform.

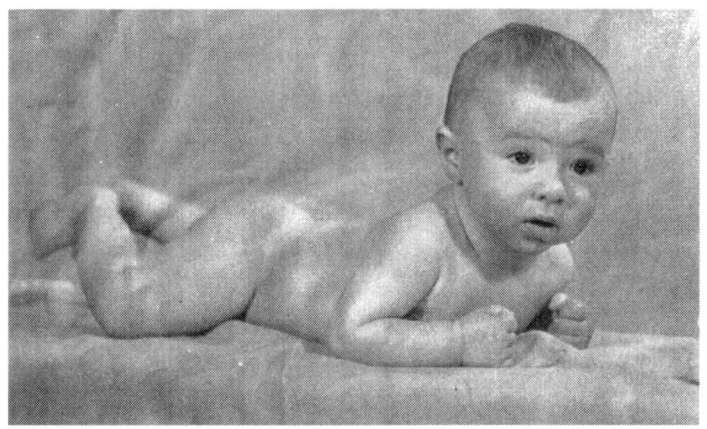

Ed as a baby.

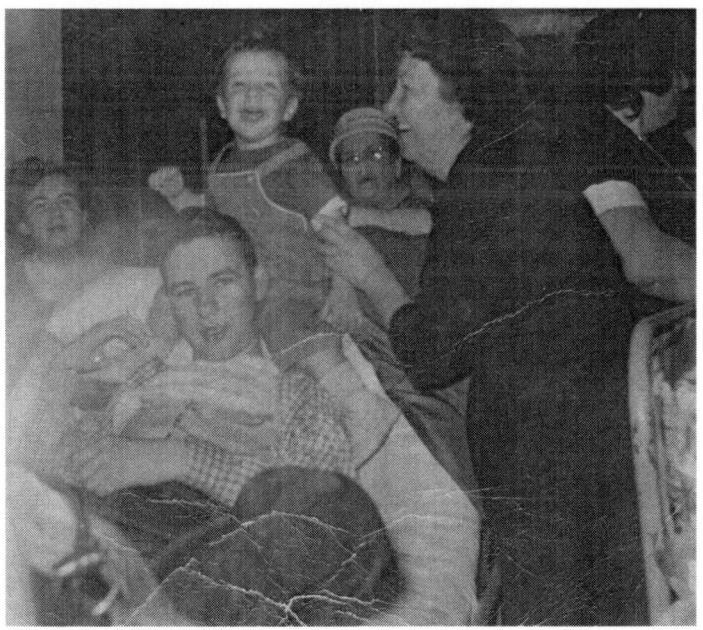

Ed at Sunnyview Rehab with his mom and siblings.

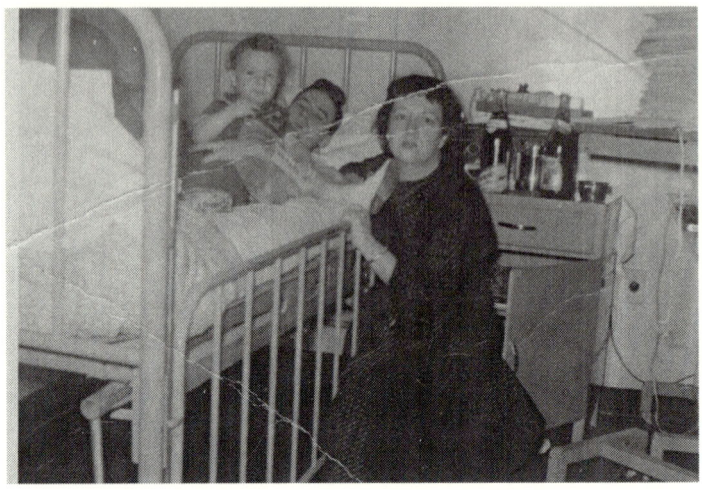
Ed with his brother "Feather" and their mom.

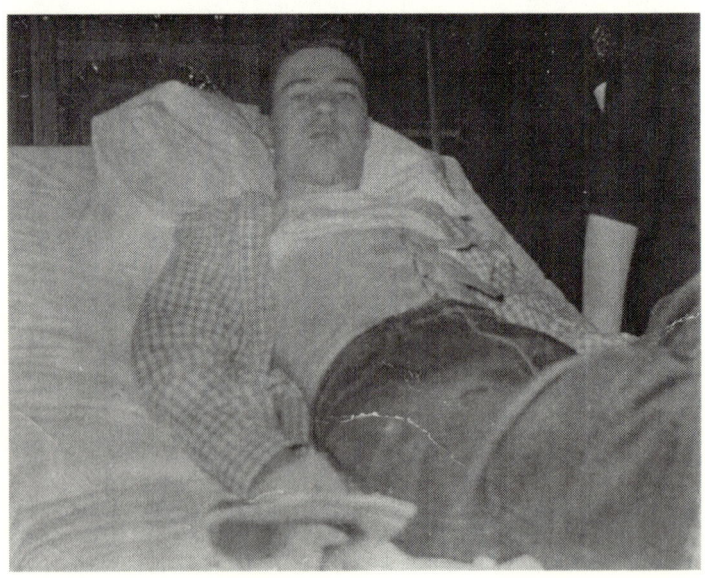
Ed's back brace is visible.

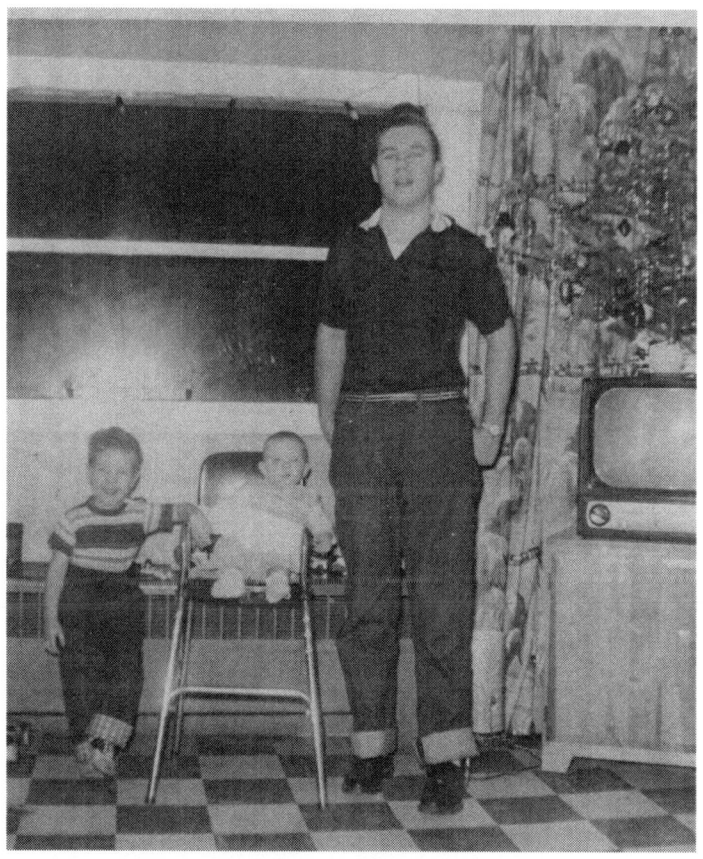

Ed back at home with his brace. On the left, Feather and Pat.

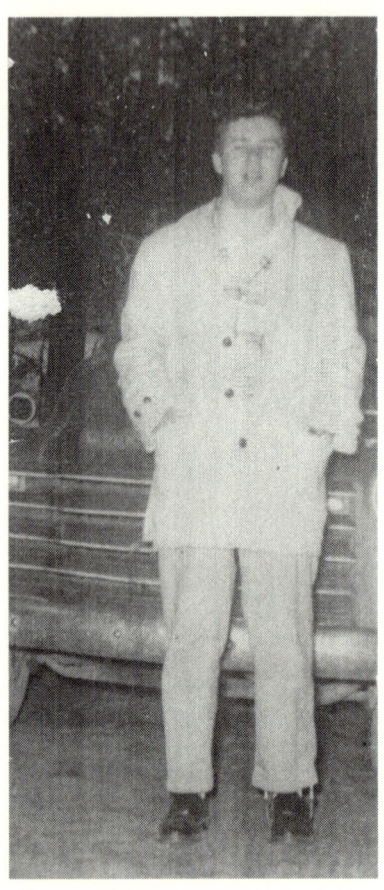

Ed standing tall after returning from Sunnyview.

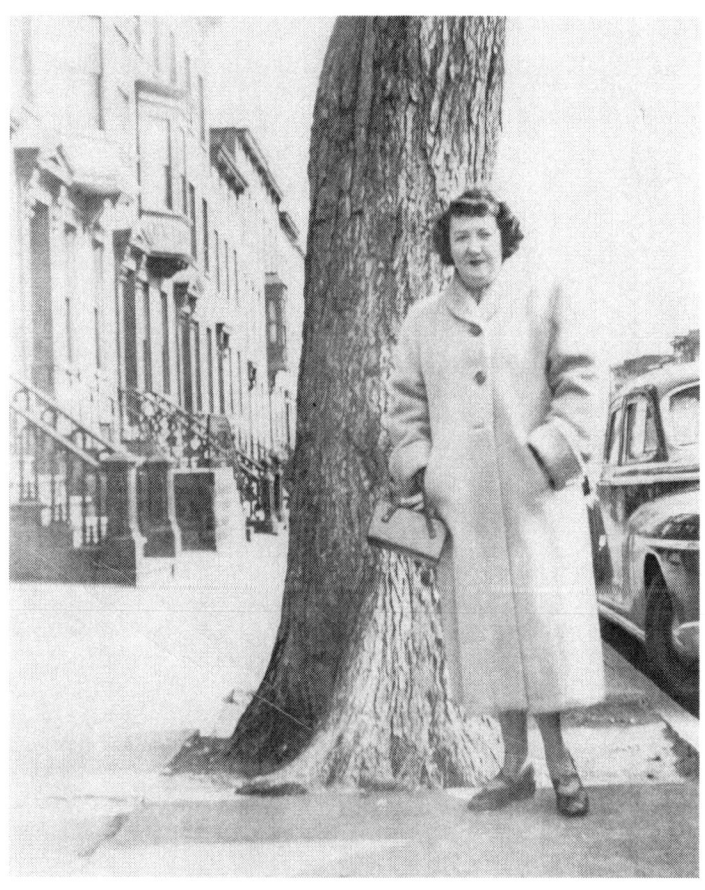

Irene Sill (Ed's mom) in front of their home in Albany.

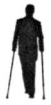

Back to High School

Friends Forever

Bobby Webber, a neighbor, ended up becoming a close buddy of mine, a lifelong friend, but we had to duke it out first. We had a disagreement when we were teenagers and had a knockdown, bloody-nose fight and after that we were friends. We were in each other's weddings and have kept in touch all these years. Our family and his family would do a lot together through the years. Bob died from pancreatic cancer at the age of sixty-four.

My other friends in the neighborhood were Eddie and Arnie Godfrey. Eddie had a "22" rifle and he used to bring it up to my house, on the hill. We had several places on the hill where we could shoot a rifle safely. One was a partially dug out swimming pool area and because it had a sand pit backing we used to place targets in the bottom of the 4-foot end. We would shoot guns there and one day we happened to miss. We shot a 22 that had what they called long rifle shots in it at the time. As you might guess, the bullet carried into a new development in the rear of our property about a half a mile away and it went right through somebody's picture window and hit a wall. Luckily, it didn't hurt anybody but it certainly could have killed someone. The state troopers were called. The troopers went to the surrounding houses and hills and tried to figure out where the bullet had come from. One trooper came up to our house. We went outside and he asked us if we knew anything about any shootings. Naturally, at the time, we played dumb and told him we weren't aware of any shooting. Actually, it is a good thing that the trooper did not look down on the ground, and it was hard to believe that he did not roll on some of the bullet casings when he walked around the property, because we did not clean up our mess after shooting the gun. It would have been certainly an easy thing to spot but luckily someone was watching over us and things worked out okay.

Two other people in the neighborhood played an important role in my life. One was Bob Snyder, who lived about a mile away, another lifelong friend. He had quit school in the 11th grade at Guilderland Central. On the days I would have trouble getting Mrs. Trager to pick me up and go to Albany Medical Center for my physical therapy or rehabilitation, Bob would take me. He had a driver's license and a truck and would take me down for my treatments. He threw me around like a brother and handled me in and out of his truck along with the Canadian crutches. It was always nice to have a helping hand whenever I had to go for these treatments. Although several of our friends have died, Bob and I still keep in touch.

Another boyhood chum was Bruce Perry. Bruce and I were schoolmates too. He was a funny type kid; he lived on Church Road, about a quarter of a mile away. His father raised pigs and livestock so it was somewhat of a farm atmosphere there. One time in particular, I remember going up to his house to play. We used to do a lot of things together, build tree forts and different things of that nature, baseball, run the bases, kill-the-carrier in football and all kinds of fun things.

Bruce was the type of kid who wanted to prove that he could beat you up; he tried that with me several times, for what reason I don't know. But he never did come out on top, as I always seemed to beat him in wrestling, boxing, or whatever sport we were involved in. One day we got a real rude awaking. His father had been in the service years before and owned an Army "45" pistol. He invited us to go up to the area where they raised some pigs and other animals and he actually took the 45 pistol and shot two of the pigs several times through the head to kill them for slaughter. He had the talent to take care of his own meat and butcher and freeze it. Boy, what a shock that was to a young kid to hear how loud a 45 pistol would shoot and how it could take down an animal with two or three bullets; that was quite a surprise.

Bruce was also in trouble several times in school at Guilderland. Another funny story on him—he always like to go against the grain. Every Friday we had what was called "Dress up Day." One day Bruce decided to wear red—red band pants that you would wear in a band competition. Boy, at the time, that was just not allowed. You talk about funny times in different eras, what is accepted and what isn't. Well, the teachers and the principal were so upset about his dress that day that they sent him home to change his clothes or not to come back to school that day. Well, I guess he chose not to come back to school so his father had to come up and see the principal a week later to get him back in school.

Another funny memory was a kid we called "Preacher Right." At the time, a lot of people were becoming aware of not only religious things but they were trying to tune themselves with nature. This boy had a bad habit of eating caterpillars off the trees and preaching to everybody and trying to get people to come around to his religious beliefs which were pretty far-fetched at the time so we really didn't put much stock in Preacher Right. It seemed so incongruous that somebody trying to preach to you would eat caterpillars off the tree limbs in the rear of the school where the athletic field was. Once again, in high school you never know what's going to happen so you just kind of ride the tide.

We used to go to Bobby Webber's house before we would go to dances at the high school. There again, boyhood mischief came into play. We would all take a swig off the wine bottle so we would have enough nerve to ask girls to dance with us. It was always the same old four guys hanging around and getting into trouble together. I won't get into all of it now, but I will say that you learn a lot in your teenage years that really sticks with you for the rest of your life. As the story progresses, I think a lot of that will come into being.

Also, during this time I learned another valuable lesson—never fight over a girl. We had an occasion where Hilton Holzhauer and I were in a class and we both liked a girl named Mary Ann Simone. Well, you might know, we had words one day in class and we started fighting and I smacked Hilton pretty good and he went flying up against the blackboard and sunk down to the floor and was stunned for a couple of seconds. Actually, I may have come out on the wrong end of that one because I broke my thumb. I guess it didn't pay to fight over a girl and it ended up as the same old story, neither one of us wound up with the girl. She ended up with a basketball player named Billy Norton.

First Girlfriends

Baseball and sports were fun, but now I was becoming interested in better school grades, cars, travel, and dating girls. One of my first loves in high school was a cheerleader named Mary Ann Simone. She was a very good-looking girl, and was in a lot of my classes. We would tease each other about silly things like bringing a ladder up to her house window and maybe eloping. You know just boy and girl fun talk and a little on the serious side but mostly on the kidding side.

The second girl I took out was Lynn Eisley. She was older than I was, in the 11th grade when I was in the 9th. She was kind of a tomboy, who liked to wrestle with the boys and twist your fingers until you would say "uncle." She tried to prove that she was tougher than the boy she was going out with, I guess. Actually, it got to be tiresome after awhile. We used to double-date; a friend of mine had a car and traveled to Guilderland Center to take some girls out and would usually walk quite a way around the streets where Lynn lived and would usually wind up in a wrestling match. After awhile, I kind of got tired of the tomboy girl act and decided to move around and see who else was available.

The next girl that I was interested in was Judy Fowler. Judy was a very nice looking blonde, also in a lot of my classes, about my age and we used to have a lot of fun hanging out and going to dances. I don't know what happened, but you know how young adolescents are, it was time to find another girlfriend. So I started going out with a girl from Altamont, named Andrea Ross, she was (once again) older than I was and she was going to graduate a year or two ahead of me so I didn't see too much future in that relationship. Once again it was time to move on.

I started taking out a pretty redhead girl named Rhonda. Usually I double-dated with Bobby Snyder and his girl (he had several). After we went out on a date, we could home and have a cigarette and hash over how our dates went and what we learned and what we didn't learn about the girls we took out and what we were interested in. We both came to the same conclusion. If you dated a girl three times and you weren't going anywhere, then it was either time to move on or ask her to go steady with you. When I was taking Rhonda out and we had about three or four dates, I figured it was time to ask her if we were going to be more of item than just friends and asked if she would like to go steady. She said, "Well, I probably would, because I like you a lot, but I am engaged to a Marine and when he comes home from the service this June, we plan to get married." Boy, did that startle me! I was surprised at that. So, you find out early in life that love is a game and yet it's fun and has its trials and tribulations, just like anything else. After the Rhonda episode, I decided that I would not be so eager and quick to give my heart away and also look for romance or put too much pressure on anybody. Actually, that was a better idea for someone between 16 and 18 years of age.

    I started hanging around with several friends who had cars: Archie Haughton, Ritchie Drowne, Bobby Snyder, Al Austin, and Bobby Webber. Most of these guys were at the age to get their driving permit or license. It was time to get into more teenage mischief. Several of us had copies of someone's driver's license. He would claim to have lost his license and would go down to the Motor Vehicle Department and get a duplicate copy without too much problem. We all had a license and would all claim to be this guy for identity purposes and also being able to drive a car. We all felt we needed a license because we spent a lot of time at the Happy Day Nursery on Friday nights to go dancing. It was kind of a teenage hangout on the weekends and a lot of fun. It was on Schoolhouse Road in Westmere. Everybody and their brother would go there on the weekends and it was just a lot of fun. It had good music, mostly a disc jockey with records but later on they brought in live bands. We all had a good time there. The Kennedy Building was another dance hall we used to go to on weekends.

Ed Meets Sandie

When my friends Archie Haughton and Ritchie Drowne went to a birthday party and met some new girls, Archie said, "Ed I think you should meet this girl, Sandie. I think you would like her." I kind of foo-fooed it at the time, but later said, "Well, maybe I should meet this girl."

Archie at the time had a 1950 Ford convertible. That was a funny story too. We tried to repaint his car and it didn't come out very good. It was a lemon-colored car when he first got it, had to do a lot of work on it to repair it, and we wound up painting it black. Anyway, we had wheels. We went over to Rensselaer, across the bridge from Albany. There I met Sandie LaMountain. We started dating, going to Lebanon Valley Stock Car Races, danced, did a lot of things teens like to do. We went to state parks, swimming and always had a good time together. Soon we became more than friends, started going steady and had a lot of fun together. I guess you always wonder whether these things will someday lead to marriage or whether it will go nowhere because you do date so many people in the teenage years. But as things worked out, we wound up getting married. I was 20 years old and Sandie was 18.

Our first home was a mobile home that my father owned on Church Road, so we weren't very far from the family. My mother and father lived on top of the hill and on the bottom of the hill was a big sand bank where the mobile home was. We lived here when we first got married and when we had our first child, Tammy Marie. We were kind of young but knew what direction we wanted to go in. At the time I was driving a 1958 Plymouth, but when we first got married I had a 1955 Chevy. It really proved to be a real lemon, it was white and yellow. My father had advised me not to buy it as it had a lot of problems, including motor problems, the lifters were all messed up but you know how teenagers are, they don't want to listen to their parents. They want to find their own independence. Well, I bought the car and certainly made a mistake, because I was putting more money into the car than anything else we were doing. It was mounting up to the point that I had to get rid of it and ended up trading it in for the Plymouth and that wound up being a really super car.

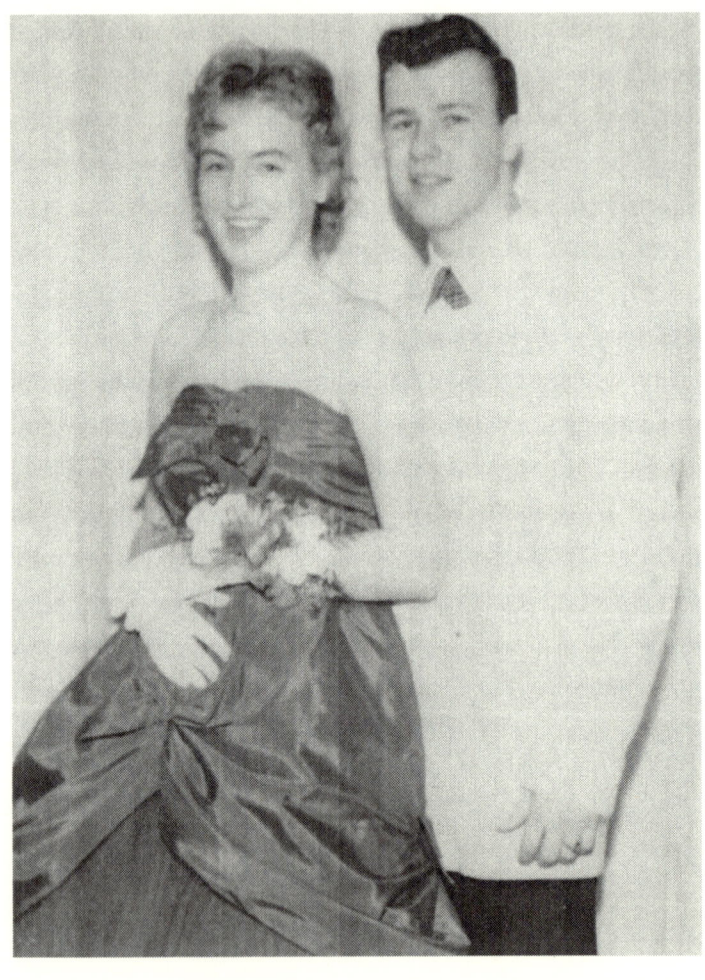

Sandie and Ed at her senior prom.

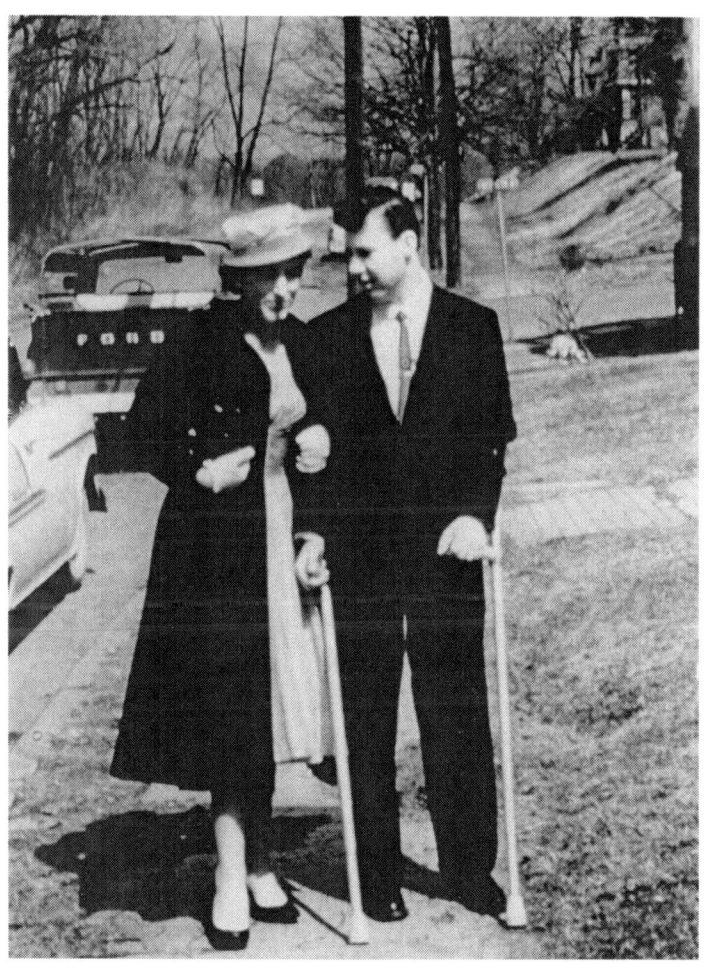

Sandie and Ed on Easter Sunday, 1960.

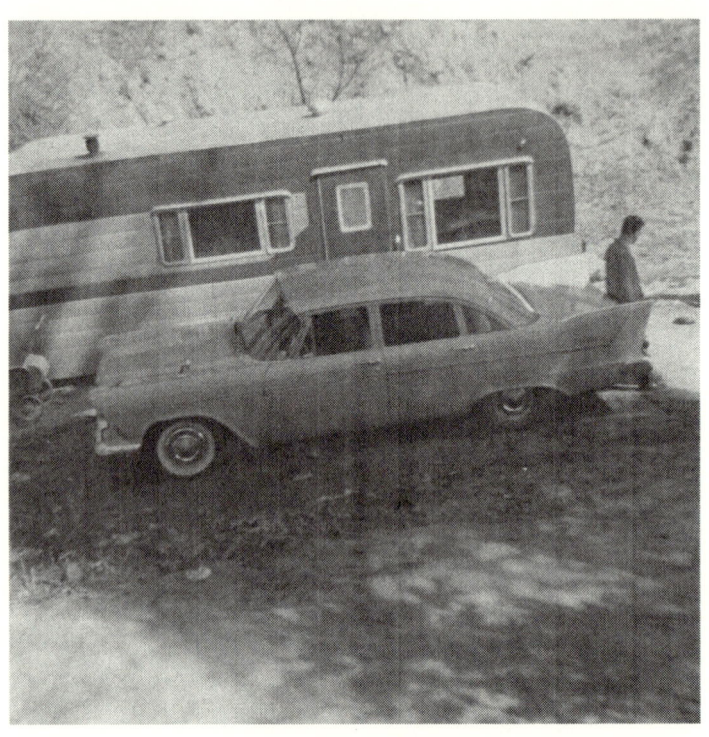

Sandie and Ed's first home and car.

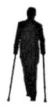

Sandie Meets Ed

*This is where Ed's tape ended, so I will
continue our story from here
—Sandie*

Sandie Remembers

It was my 16th birthday party. My infatuation that day was with a boy named Joey. He was interested in my girlfriend Joan. I was following him around while he was following Joan. After awhile someone said a car pulled up with a bunch of guys in it. I went out front and there was Artie, a friend of Joey's. He introduced me and the others to the guys and most of them were out of the car. But one guy, who was pretty darn cute, was just talking to us from the car and he kept directing questions to me. After talking to him for awhile I asked him if he was anti-social, because he wasn't getting out of the car. He said "no, if you want I'll get out." Then he opened the door and "clunked" his two leg braces out of the car door. He had two leg braces on and a back brace. I was so embarrassed for saying something to him, now realizing he was handicapped. I apologized and of course, he took advantage of my blunder by saying, "Well if you're sorry, then you have to go out on a date with me." I said I would (as I thought he was real handsome), but was actually a bit nervous, as I didn't know what to expect. He was easy to talk to and we started to see each other a lot. After a summer at his cousin's campgrounds where he could swim every day, he lost the back brace and one leg brace. He was doing much better.

We called each other every night and talked. He didn't have a car at first, so if we went anywhere we had to go with one of his buddies who had a car or they would drop him off at my house and pick him up later. My family loved to play card games and one of the games was pinochle. He had never played it and wanted to learn it. So we taught him how to play and he was addicted, so every time he was over we had to play pinochle.

One of our weekend events was going to the stock car racetrack at Lebanon Valley. We would get a bunch of us together and bring our blankets because it was usually pretty cool there. There was always a certain car we liked and rooted for. That was a lot of fun. We went to a lot of the dances in the area, at my school, Happy Day Nursery or the Kennedy Building. Surprisingly he tried to keep up with me. I loved to dance and he knew it so he would do his best to get out there and try it. Ed was now down to one leg brace and able to balance much better. He and his buddy wanted dancing lessons, so we went to the basement of his home and put the 45s on and I would try to show them how to dance. It was challenging, but fun.

The amazing thing about Ed was that when we went to the dance halls all these guys with good legs would be standing there checking out the girls and here is this guy who is challenged with a leg brace and he would be out there jitterbugging with me. I always gave him so much credit for doing that and he earned respect from a lot of people. And we had some pretty sexy waltzes too.

In the wintertime, dating was interesting, as Ed lived on the top of a hill. When it was snowy or icy, his buddy would come and pick me up first. He would park the car at the bottom of the hill and climb up the hill, put Ed on a sled and push him down on the sled. I would catch him at the bottom of the hill and his buddy would come down, put him in the car and off we would go to pick up his buddy's girlfriend and go to our destination. When he couldn't maneuver in the snow, his buddies were great — they would throw him around like a sack of potatoes, in and out of the car or carry him to the building where we were going. The friends we had then, we still have now. They are great people and we have so many good memories of all the fun we had, like the popcorn fights at the local drive-in theaters in Artie's convertible and the parties at Marion and Helene's house.

Tying the Knot

We broke up a couple of times and ended up back together. We went together for about two and a half years, off and on before we decided to get married.

We got married in 1961 at St. Joseph's Church in Rensselaer and one of Ed's buddies, John Puspurs, offered to be the DJ. For our music, all our friends got together their 45s and he played them at a little church hall up the hill from the church we were married in. The food was catered by the families, and everyone brought something.

Right out of High School, Ed applied for a clerk position at Sterling Winthrop Research Institute in Rensselaer and was hired. His brother-in-law, Jerry, worked there and had let him know that there were a few openings available. He really liked the job and, over the years, became so good at memorizing the file numbers of each of the products they sold or researched that when someone would ask about a product, he would recite the file number off the top of his head. It wasn't a high paying position but there was chance for advancement and I was also working as a stenographer for an electrical contractor, so we could manage. We rented the trailer, which his parents owned, and it was at the bottom of the hill from their home. It was small but worked for us then. We would have to look for something else as the family grew.

Our life got busy right away after our marriage as we had our new baby, Tammy. I was not working right after Tammy was born and was watching my sister-in-law, Patty, who was about 4 years old, for his mom when she was at her job. Almost a year later, we had news that I was pregnant again. So looking for a bigger home was going to be on our list of things to do.

We had to move from the trailer quicker than we were planning, since his parents were getting a divorce and things were getting ugly. We literally took all our belongings one night and had to stay at my aunt's home for a couple of nights. We could not find a place to rent that fast and I certainly would not be able to move us in my condition. One of our friends asked if they could help and offered to put us up until the baby was born. We took them up on the offer and Ronald Edward was born a few weeks later.

A Close Call

We had a close call with the baby while we were there. The bassinet we borrowed had a mattress that was a little larger than it should be and went up on the sides. I had put him down on his belly for a nap and when I went to check him I noticed he looked very pale. I picked him up and noticed he wasn't breathing so I performed CPR on him and, thank God, his breathing came back. What a scare that was and I never put him on his belly again! The Lord was with me that day because I had only put him down a little while and usually didn't check on him that soon.

After a few weeks, we knew we needed to move out of our friend's home as soon as possible to give them their home back. I can never thank them enough for being so kind to put up with us for the time they did. It was a big sacrifice to have to deal with a new emotional mother, a handicapped man and two babies when they only had one child of their own. We were having trouble finding a place that would take children. So we packed up what we could and went up to my mother's home, which was an apartment in Whitehall, two hours away, until we could find something local. Ed would come up on the weekends to visit and go back on Sunday nights to get ready for work. He was staying at his oldest sister Rena's home in Albany during the workweek.

My sister found a place in Schenectady that we might be able to get. It was on the second floor though, so I was skeptical as to how Ed would get up and down the stairs. He wasn't worried, he said he could scoot himself up the stairs on his behind if he needed to. So we rented it, as there didn't seem to be many options at the time. It was quite a ride for him to go to work as he worked in Rensselaer, about 25 miles away. We were trying to save some money for a down payment on a house nearer his work, which was a big struggle in those days because we usually lived from paycheck to paycheck and there was not a lot left over. God bless Ed, even though we fought about it sometimes, he managed to save a little each time for our goal.

I was rushed to the hospital one day for pains in my abdomen and after operating and removing my appendix, the doctor smiled and said, "Congratulations Mom, you're going to have a baby". Another child, Kenneth Robert, was born nine months later.

We lived with some crates and kitchen chairs in the living room for awhile until we could afford a living room couch and chair. I ran to the Laundromat to wash and dry clothes and diapers. We did manage to buy a washing machine after Ken was born, hung clothes on the line off the porch to dry. Yes, we had cloth diapers in those days. There were diaper services that would take the pail of diapers, wash, dry and bring them back for you if you could afford that.

Ed would scoot up and down the stairs twice a day to get to his car and drive back and forth to work. Another year passed after Kenny was born and I found out I was pregnant again. Now with two small bedrooms, where would we put another baby? It was already crowded, so we decided to push harder to save that down payment money. Finally, we got together $500, a lot of money in the 60s, and put it down on a two-story home in Rensselaer, which was about a mile or so away from Ed's work. We moved in the fall of 1965 and I was due around Thanksgiving for our fourth child. We lived in a small city now, where I grew up. I was thrilled to have a home of our own because my family never owned a home. Ed was very proud to be able to provide one for his family.

Our New Home

We moved in August and I was due in November around Thanksgiving. Ed's friends and my relatives all got together and moved us. We were so excited to have bedrooms for the kids and breathing room for us all. Our yard was small but fenced in so the kids could go out in the yard to play. It was comfortable for us. We ended up living there for 28 years.

To get up the stairs at night, Ed would have me bring the crutches up to the top of the stairs (as the kids got older, this was their job) and he would scoot up those stairs and get up on his crutches and walk or scoot to the bed. His arms were very strong and powerful. He could get up from the floor with one crutch—it was amazing the strength he had in those arms.

In October, Ed fell in the dining room and broke his leg. Well, strong as I was dealing with three toddlers and a big belly, this was a lot on my emotional stamina. Ed had a cast on and couldn't get around much, so it was "San, could you get me this?" And then the kids would be pulling at me to do something or fighting over a toy. Our best man's wife, Diane, offered to stay with our kids and Ed, when I went in to have the fourth baby. My family was not around the area and I was due around Thanksgiving, so they gave up their family outing to stay around in case I went to have the baby. Well it was not to be, for Turkey Day. Our new baby girl, Denise Irene, came a few weeks late and she was born December 4th. They had a little boy of their own, so God bless them for being there for us at the time and taking in three more toddlers and a handicapped man for a week. At home, we had no dryer so had to hang clothes in the cellar to dry, even the diapers. I remember crying a lot that year and praying to God saying, "Knowing that you only give us as much as we can handle, please know that this is it, I can't handle anymore!"

So now we had the family we wanted, very happy that God

had blessed us with two boys and two girls. How lucky can we get?

Ed was doing well at work and getting regular salary raises. Things were getting busy when the children got into programs at school, etc. Our kids were so much fun and soooo smart, "smarter than any kid around!"

When money got tight, I went to work at the local department store, part time, in walking distance of our home. When Ed came home, he got a kiss from me, dinner would be ready for everyone and I would walk out the door to work, hours were usually 5 to 9 pm.

Sportswriter

Ed also did some part-time sports writing for the GAN, an East Greenbush newspaper. Ed always had the "gift of gab" and loved his sports. An opportunity came up for sportswriter for a local paper and Ed accepted it. This job was something he would like because now he would have to go to the local games and report on them and get some feedback from the locals. He loved talking and met a whole different group of people from the area. He enjoyed it until it got to be too hard to keep up with it all (work, family time and sports writing).

Mark Rozell

Ed liked helping the neighborhood kids, especially the ones who didn't have a father around. One of the neighborhood boys was Mark Rozell. He was a "special needs" child, but very smart and very handsome. He was a very curious boy and would ask Ed all sorts of questions. Ed would answer them or even show him things so he understood. Mark was little when he would see Ed walk by his house. Mark and his mother Theresa would talk to Ed. When he was old enough to come to the house by himself, he would go for a walk with Ed and Ed would have him pick up the litter on their way around the block. Mark never minded helping and he would say, "We're cleaning up the city, huh Ed?" Ed would say "you bet, you're doing a great job, Mark!" He was just a sweetheart of a kid, but the kids in school would just tease him something terrible. Mark ended up getting ready to graduate at age 19, and was so excited. He was in the Key Club and had gone on a weekend with them before graduation and when he came home he said to his mom that he wasn't feeling well and went and laid down for awhile. He just didn't feel good. He never got up and passed away in his sleep.

A newspaper article, "School memories of Mark Rozell endure beyond his death," talked about how he was injured in an auto accident. He seemed alright and even donated blood when the Key Club sponsored a blood drive. Three days later, when he returned home from a Key Club Convention, he told his mom he was not feeling good and she later found him dead in his bed. His mom talked about when he was younger, they called him "retarded" and how today they call him a "saint". The article reviewed Mark's accomplishments and all of the good things he did through his life. The school said that awards in his name will continue to do good for others. One of his teachers, Mike Fusco Jr., said that Mark never used profane words and that the only four-letter word Mark knew was "love."

The city was devastated, especially the kids who picked on him for years, since he didn't make it to his graduation. At the graduation ceremony everyone cried when they mentioned his name. Ed and I and our family were a mess, because it was like part of our family died. He will always be in our hearts. Ed and Mark are surely taking walks together again now.

Ed was usually out on the front porch after work and always on the weekends when the weather was nice. He loved to talk and got to know all the neighbors well and talked to anyone that went by the house. Our home was on one of the side streets that went to the local department store in town and people would go by and beep their horns. So he was well known in the city. Taking a walk at night around the block helped him to visit with everyone along the way. We joined the local firehouse and enjoyed being a part of the community and met a lot of great people through the get-togethers there. Ed was Secretary at one point and had a lot of fun with the guys that he met there.

Our neighborhood is another whole story, which I won't get into now, but they were all great people and very helpful when things were tough. We had a lot of fun times and great memories there.

Ed the Politician

In 1984, Ed got into politics when one of the aldermen passed away, and he was asked to replace him. He ran for office in the next election and won. Now into politics, he was enjoying it. Re-elected for several terms after this, he put his all into helping people. Not everyone was happy with some of the decisions that had to be made with new developments at city hall, but he did try very hard to do what he thought was the right thing. He fought hard for their wants and sometimes he won the argument and sometimes he lost. But no one could say that he didn't try. Some of the people who called him regularly were a little eccentric and would take up a lot of time going over and over things on the phone with him, but he was very patient with them or if he did not agree with them, he would argue the point. He had to leave that position when we later moved to Reading, Pennsylvania in 1993.

Several newspaper articles followed Ed's political career. One announced that the local Democratic Committee would back Edward R. Sill to succeed the late Donald Hunt, as First Ward Alderman.

He would run in a special election in November 1984 to fill the remainder of the term, to the end of 1985. He also said he hoped to run for a four year term the following year and thought he had a good chance of winning in the November election.

After his appointment, another article talked about Ed's

originally being from Albany but liking Rensselaer for its "small town atmosphere." He explained that while he was interested in community affairs, he never sought a political office in the past because he hadn't had time. His commitments included coaching Babe Ruth League and Little League teams, serving as Treasurer and Secretary of the men's softball and football leagues, Secretary of the local firehouse, and Chairman of the city's Youth Board. It mentioned that he had been a technical clerk with Sterling Winthrop for 25 years.

In the article, Ed said he supported the reconstruction of South Street to remove truck traffic from Riverside Avenue, adding a youth and community center in the former Fort Crailo Elementary School, developing recreational facilities at Coyne field and in general "sprucing up Ward 1." He told of receiving more than 200 calls from constituents with a variety of problems, saying, "I'm here for the people when they don't know where to go for help."

Ed was successful in the election, beating challenger Alfred Jukes for the 1st Ward Alderman position.

In a later article, Rensselaer Mayor Joseph E. Harrigan issued an appeal for residents over age 16 to apply at city hall to serve on the Rensselaer Youth Board, whose Chairman, Alderman Edward Sill said the goal was "to devise the best method of disbursing the funds at our disposal - to get the best dollar value." He said, "We've also worked to develop programs like Easter egg hunts near city hall, outdoor movies in the city hall parking lot and sponsoring roller skating programs." He described his Youth Board as "really for anyone who is interested in providing for the needs of the youth of Rensselaer."

Summers at Lake St. Catherine in Vermont

When our kids were little, we started going up to a camp in Vermont, about a two-hour drive, where my Aunt Agnes and Uncle John went every year. Uncle John's family lived in Poultney, Vermont and he would rent a camp near them. We were invited up and decided this would be a great vacation time for us. So we rented it the next year and proceeded to rent it for the next 15 years. The kids loved it, even though there was no phone, no TV, no drinking water (we had to buy it in the jugs at the store). We had no shower either, so we picked up our soap and took baths in the lake. There was no hot water so had to heat it on the stove to do dishes or wash up in the sink. We did have a small bathroom with a toilet and sink, thank goodness. The camp was very rustic so you could hear each other from the bedrooms. It had a great screened-in porch overlooking the lake and we would watch the thunderstorms in awe from there. It was on the top of a hill, so a challenge for "Big Ed," but he had no problem getting up and down. He would just throw the crutches down the hill and scoot down on his behind. There was a rowboat and with Ed's powerful arms he could row for hours and loved taking the kids fishing. They would come home with bass, perch, and sunnies and he would ready them for the grill. Sometimes we even had fish for breakfast.

We invited our friends and their families to come up. The grill would get fired up, and the cold beer, soda, lemonade and iced tea were plentiful. The horseshoes would be flying, some would be out for a boat ride or go fishing, some would be swimming and then later the games, monopoly, yahtzee, poker or pinochle cards would come out. What great fun we had with the kids running around and playing tag or catching lightning bugs. When it came to bedtime, they were usually tired enough to sleep, except when their friends were there with them, then it was a giggle fest for a few hours.

The lake itself was beautiful and spring-fed, so you could see the bottom of the lake. As they got older the girls would go out in the rowboat and check out the guys and vice-versa. No longer fishing for fish, just fishing! We would let one friend of one of the children come each year, so it wasn't so overwhelming, but a lot of fun. On the nights when the weather permitted, we would have bonfires and everyone looked forward to that and would tell stories or sing. The owner, Marge and her son, Ron would come over almost nightly to see how things were going and we would invite them to have dinner with us or sit by the bonfire. The camp has since been torn down but I still have contact with Ron, since his mom, Marge has passed away. Ron is still in the camp next door, which was renovated for his home. What wonderful memories my children and I have of the special times we spent there.

Back at Home

Our lives were busy as the boys were into basketball at the Boys Club and baseball with Little League and Babe Ruth and we were at the field at least twice a week. The girls and boys went to the Girls and Boys Club a lot, which was in walking distance of the house. Tammy wanted to be a cheerleader and was always practicing for that. Denise liked gymnastics and was into that at the Girls Club. Several different jobs were part of my life as conditions changed at the house. I started out of high school as a stenographer and had a couple of jobs in that field before the children were born. Then I cooked at the elementary school when my children were going to school there, did part-time retail sales at the local department store, taught cake decorating at Adult Ed classes, worked as a waitress at the bowling alley, worked at the governor's office doing research, as a purchasing agent for a bearing company, etc. When Ed starting getting sick I was working full time and helping my boss start a new business and became General Manager of the Construction Products Company.

When our children were young our social life consisted of getting together with friends for cards or rummy or board games most weekends. For example, Fran and Lenny's house was usually the site of a Sunday night pinochle game. We would pack up all four kids and off we'd go to someone's house, bringing blankets so the kids could sleep when they got tired. Later we would carry them back out to the car to go home. Our friends would take turns carting their kids to our house too.

Ed and I had some frustrating times and arguments about not seeing each other, as we seemed to be going in two different directions at times, so after talking about it we agreed to get out at least once a month together without the kids for some time alone. We always had a good time, since we both enjoyed music and loved to dance. Usually if there was a good band or DJ we would be one of the last to leave, so we took full advantage of our night out. We even started to follow one of the bands we liked, going to wherever they would be playing next.

That Little Old Winemaker, Ed

I remember when Ed decided he wanted to make wine. He bought one of those wine-making kits and started cutting up and saving various fruit as ingredients, which he would put in a big plastic jug on top of the refrigerator until it was time to test the wine. Some of it was pretty good, but then he started adding fruit that was not really made for wine and then it would not be so tasty. One morning I got up and discovered the whole top of the refrigerator was stripped of paint. The fermented wine was leaking and took all the paint off. We laughed at that, telling everyone that Ed made some pretty powerful wine. We told our friends that if they needed any paint thinner, he would make them some.

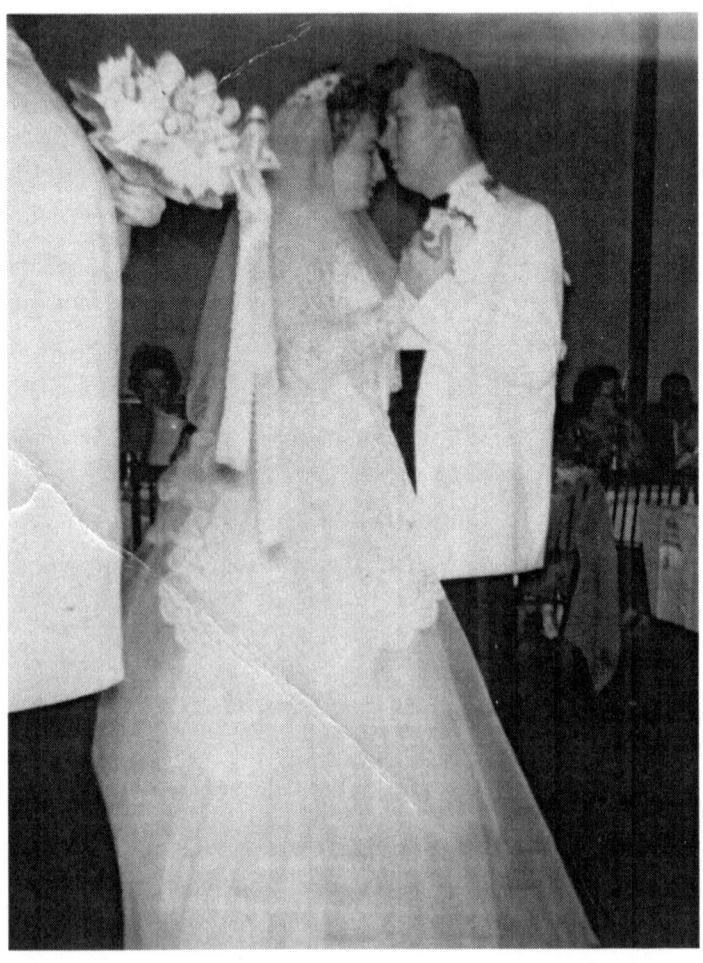

Sandie and Ed's wedding dance.

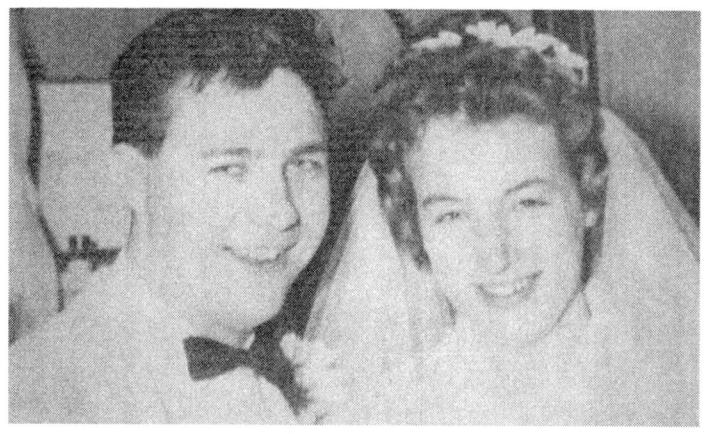

Sandie and Ed on their wedding day.

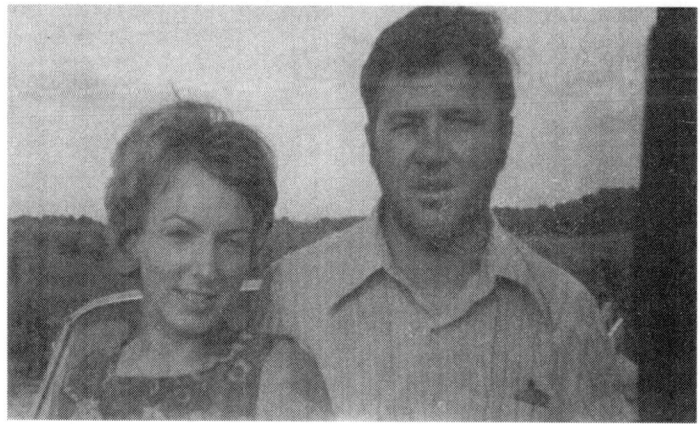

Sandie and Ed.

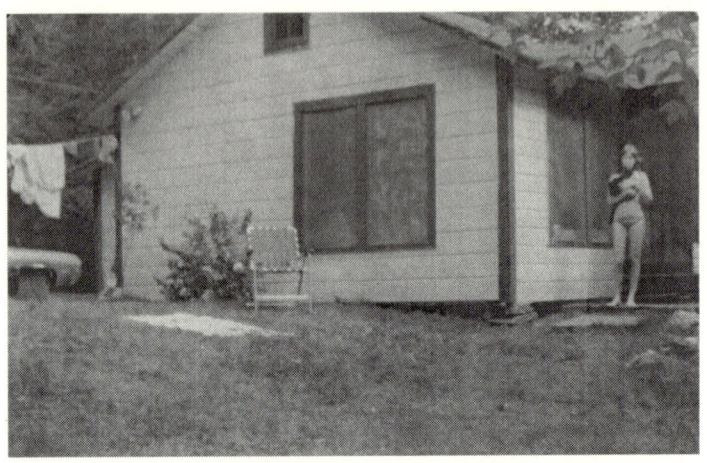

The cabin at Lake St. Catherine.

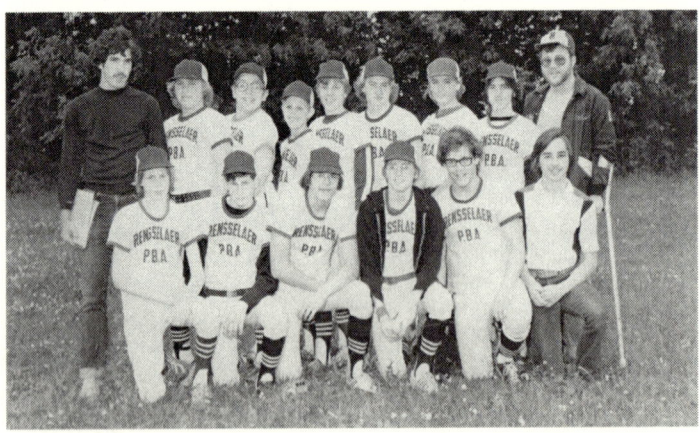

Ed and Kevin Perrotte with the Babe Ruth team they coached.

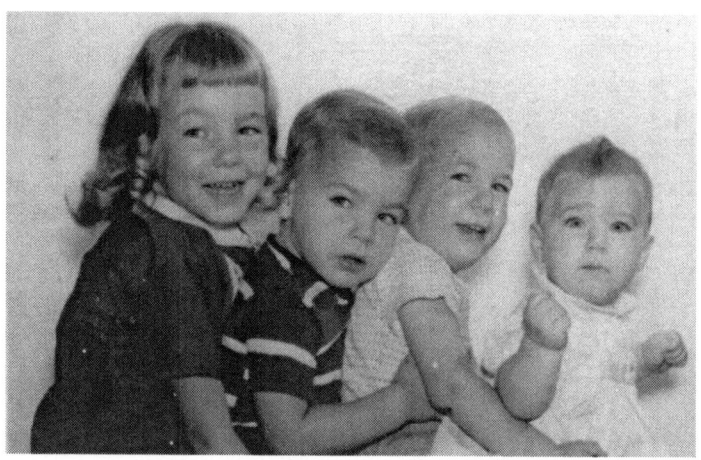

Our children when they were young: Tammy, Ron, Ken, and Denise.

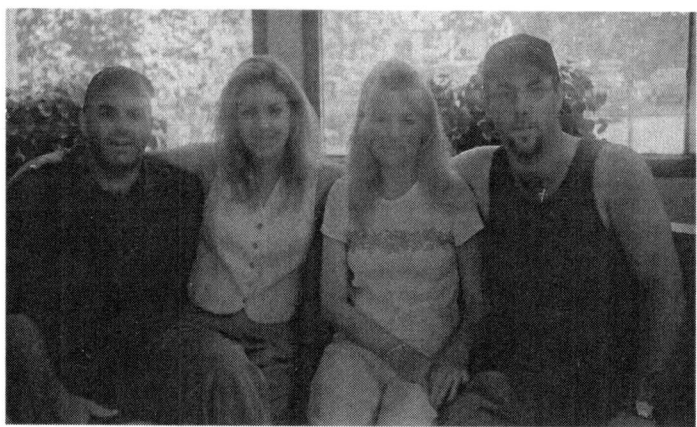

Our children as adults.

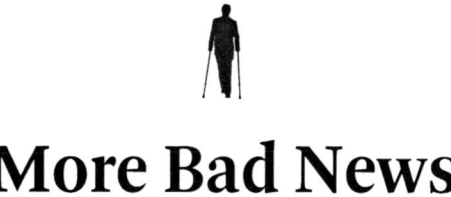

More Bad News

Ed Is Diagnosed With Cancer

Sometime in 1980 Ed had not been feeling well and seemed to be getting weaker by the day. The doctor couldn't pinpoint anything so he sent us to an orthopedic doctor to see if something was going on there. Well, this doctor was checking him out and trying to make him stand by himself without the brace. He had never been able to do that without the brace and almost fell over. He had taken an x-ray and found no broken bones, etc. We were not happy with this doctor as he seemed to insinuate that Ed was faking something and trying to get disability, which Ed never wanted to do, because he could not find out what was wrong.

We went to another doctor, who thought maybe he was having some neurological problem or that there was something going on with the polio again, but there was no resolution. He was going to do some tests but we never got back there. He had to go lay down in the nurse's office every day at work. One morning he woke up and I took one look at him and saw how yellow he looked and I said to him "we need to bring you to the hospital" and he said "No, I'm going to go to work and see what the nurse says." He was insistent on this but we both knew he was jaundiced and both of us were tired of getting the runaround with these other doctors.

As soon as he walked into work he went to the nurse's office. She called an ambulance and then called me to meet them at the hospital. His pharmaceutical company was doing some research at that hospital, so he was hoping that they would make sure he got a good doctor who knew what he was doing (that was his strategy for going to work with yellow jaundice). Well, after doing a CT scan they found out that he had a massive tumor in the stomach area and it was pressing on the liver and other vital organs. His gall bladder was also bad, so they went in and took out the gall bladder and took a biopsy of the tumor to send out for diagnosis.

They told us it might be cancer and we were devastated, because for some reason you never think it will happen to you or your family. Well, in those days, they sent out the biopsy and did not find out things as fast as they do today, we were told that it may be about one to two weeks before we could find out what they were dealing with. Ed was very ill, they were draining the bile out so he was hooked up to a bunch of things. He was losing weight rapidly and looked terrible. We talked and cried about the news and were praying and asking God for his help.

Upset with this because he was just 40 years old and too young to die, I needed to talk to someone and didn't know who the oncologist would be yet. The gastric bypass surgeon was very good with us and said if I had any questions to come and see him. One day, after waiting for some news as to what it was, I walked the halls looking for his office and crying. He brought me in to his office and we sat and talked. I asked him to please tell me what it could possibly be and what his chances were. He told me a list of cancers and whether or not they were terminal or treatable. I needed to know what we might be dealing with.

I was at Ed's side every day but did not tell him everything the doctor told me that day except that there were treatable cancers. I went home that night and cried and prayed so hard talking to God and said, "It is your decision as to whether Ed lives or dies. I'm hoping you decide to leave him here with us for awhile longer but whatever you have decided I will deal with." Then I slept for the first time in a while.

A Divine Message

When I saw Ed the next day, he pulled me close to him and whispered, "San, I saw the Lord last night!" The goosebumps went up and down me. He told me that he saw the Lord come to him with his arms open wide, but he didn't say anything. He said I don't know if that is a sign that I will live or die, but I am ready to do what he wants. I told Ed about my intensive prayer and the calmness that came over me after praying. So we had both resolved that whatever the Lord had in mind we would be able to deal with now.

Ed was never much for religion, but he did believe in God. He went to church with me on Easter and Christmas, but only occasionally went to Mass with me on Sundays. It was harder for him with the Canadian crutches to be comfortable in the pews. When I told him about a vision I had in my teens he would just give me this look, like "Sure you did!" He probably didn't believe me at the time, but I knew now he believed that it happened.

The results of the biopsy came back and it was diagnosed as non-Hodgkin's lymphoma. The type he had was treatable. There was a teaching doctor at the hospital, Dr. Spears, who was amazing and did a lot to keep Ed going and alive. He was trying a new treatment and they explained what it involved and Ed said "go for it." He had to stay at the hospital for awhile, just healing from the gall bladder operation. Then they started the treatment and he was able to come home and do it on an out-patient basis. He would have projectile vomiting and did not want to take any of the anti-nausea meds as he thought they would make him light headed and not be able to walk on his crutches. He did give in to some of it after quite a few bouts of projectile vomiting. The treatments were rough in those days, as they did not have the doses figured out yet and did not have the meds for anti-nausea that they have today, but it was working and taking the tumor down. He also had to go for radiation treatments for several weeks. When people asked how he was doing it was always, "I'm G-R-E-A-T!" After that treatment, he went a few years and had another bout. Now it was in his groin area.

Several years later, there was another bout or recurrence. His remissions would be anywhere from one to four years. Sometimes he had to be out on disability as he was unable to work. Some of the treatments were milder than others and he would be able to go back to work, even if it was part-time. One of the treatments that he had was horrible. It is a wonder that he survived the treatment. It involved Ed taking a very large number of prednisone tablets (all at once) and I had to give him a shot every day for the antidote. He would just crawl into bed and say "leave me alone." Wouldn't talk to anyone and didn't even want me around.

The family was devastated, as this was not Ed. He was close to having a breakdown and so was I. Seeing him in this condition was so hard for all of us; I cried a lot then and so did our children. But he pulled out of that one also... remarkable! The thing that we noticed with cancer, was that after several times of going through this, you just never get used to hearing that word. Every time we would go back to the doctor's office for a report we would think that we could handle it if he said it was back again, but, guess what, your heart sinks again and the tears come down when they say, "we found a new tumor." Here we go again... we would take a deep breath... and pray for God to give us the strength to deal with another bout.

In-between all these treatments Ed kept active with the community, along with his Alderman work. He was president of the Babe Ruth League, and still tried to get the kids over to the field to play sandlot ball and take them fishing when he could. At one time he also was manager of a softball team at Coyne Field, and tried to keep up with the football league when that was going on. I look back and don't know how we kept up with it all. But we were not bored... and had lots of friends that we loved being with. They were very supportive and helpful.

We Move to Pennsylvania

Ed's company, Sterling Winthrop, was being bought out by Kodak and he was offered an upgrade to move to Collegeville, Pennsylvania, where a new plant was being built. The Rensselaer Research Division was being dispersed. It was a big decision for us as we had lived there for 28 years, but we were both ready for a change. All of our children were on their own now and our animals had both passed away. The area where the company moved was a little pricey for our salaries, but we had friends that had been down there for a while and advised which counties were a little cheaper to live in.

A July 1993 newspaper article was headlined "Rensselaer alderman steps down." It told the story of how Edward Sill had been battling cancer for 12 years, but he was determined not to let the disease stop his life.

Listing his various roles (President of Babe Ruth, Youth Board Director, etc.) it said, "Sill stepped down from the council Wednesday, because he must relocate to Pennsylvania for a job at Sterling Winthrop. "I'm certainly going to miss it", he said. "All the aldermen for the last five years have been very close. We've been like a team."

Sill said the council would probably appoint Bonnie Hahn as his successor, someone "who will look out for the people." The article explained that Sill, 53, was appointed in 1984 to succeed Donald Hunt, saying that he then ran for two more terms, winning the first race against an opponent and winning the second one uncontested.

It said that during the past year, Sill had fought his fourth bout with cancer. Although it had been difficult for him to get to meetings, the article said that he kept abreast of activities through fellow aldermen, and continued to try to help constituents, his favorite part of the job. "It was natural with me," he said. "I loved helping the people cut through the red tape. I tried to give them a hand and do whatever I could to solve their problems."

We ended up in Reading, Pennsylvania (in Exeter Township), in a lovely ranch that was much more handicap accessible then our previous home. It was about a 45-minute ride to work though, but Ed found some of the people living in the area and they all carpooled. This worked out much better for him in the years ahead because of the cancer treatments as it got to a point where he was having trouble driving at all.

We loved the new house in a nice development and our new neighbors were very nice. Family and friends got together and helped to make a ramp for Ed, as the step getting into the home was a little bit high but otherwise everything was easily accessed. Later on, as his condition changed, we had to make more changes, like a handicap toilet and a wider doorway to the bathroom.

When his company moved to Collegeville, he was in the middle of a treatment. Recommended by one of the doctors in Albany was a wonderful doctor in Paoli, a town near his work, Dr. Stephen Fox, who in Ed's words "saved my life at least ten times." He would be going to his office for outpatient chemo therapy for several different bouts or recurrences and what an amazing doctor he was. Ed and I felt comfortable with him right away, he always seemed to calm Ed down about any questions or worries he had and I do remember him telling Ed at one time, that he probably would not die of cancer because of so many new treatments coming out.

The nurses there were "angels," such caring and wonderful hearts they had with all the cancer patients. No matter what the complaint was, they would help to make you feel better or comfortable. We could never thank them enough for all their help and patience. They would even dress up for certain holidays and tell the patients to dress up for it too, always trying to keep things brighter no matter what their prognosis. No matter how Ed felt that day, he would have me dress him up with something if it was a holiday.

He went a few more years in remission and then had another bout when they found a tumor in his good leg, which put him in a wheelchair. That one made him depressed for awhile, but he would bounce back. He was working while going through the treatments. The hospital where he got his radiation was near work, but an hour from home. The office people pooled together and offered to take turns every day, taking him from work to the hospital for his radiation treatments, which were daily for several weeks. What a great group of caring people he worked for! They were so upbeat and kept him laughing, even though it was a tough time for him. The hospital gave the company a plaque for their role in helping Ed.

The group he worked for just loved him and he loved them so much that even when he should have left work, he didn't want to. His hands were numb and cold all the time so he wore gloves even in the summertime. I tried to convince him that he should probably stop working, as he was in the wheelchair full time and having a hard time doing things, but he insisted that they didn't mind helping him. He would have to go the bathroom and advise someone in the office that he was going there and to meet him in the bathroom in about five or ten minutes so they could help pull his pants up. Sometimes he would be in there for awhile, as someone would forget to go get him and he would just ask the next person who came in the door. People don't mind helping when you need it.

When someone would ask how he was and he would say, "I'm G-R-R-R-E-A-T!" or "FANNNTASTIC!" One of the worst bouts was the one in his chest area, which made him loose his breath and cough up phlegm. That one was intense and he thought he was not going to make it. It was a different type and more aggressive. He was in the hospital a lot with it.

One time, his "miracle" doctor, who had gotten him through many bouts so far, was talking to Ed, mentioning that his father was in the hospital room down the hall and was very down. Ed had me put him in the wheelchair and bring him down to meet the doctor's dad and see if he could cheer him up. The doctor thanked him and said his father was impressed that someone who had gone through as much as Ed had taken the time to come and try to cheer him up.

After this bout, the doctor had him come back every six months to get Rituxin treatments to keep it away. That seemed to be helping, but Ed was having a lot of problems with his hands; he was loosing muscle and couldn't write well anymore. We went to another doctor to see if it was carpal tunnel syndrome, and this doctor said it was and scheduled an operation for it, but he did not seem to get any better from the operation. In fact, we thought it was worse. He was having trouble with his bowels and just overall not feeling well. We were struggling to get him onto the toilet and into the bed. He recruited the neighbors to help me with him. One day he was going down the sidewalk with his wheelchair and he got all the neighbors phone numbers and put them on a list so I could call them if I needed them. He asked several of them to come over to the house to learn how to use the Hoyer Lift we had, to get him into the bed.

Ed the Investor

Ed started dabbling in the stock market, watching the market ups and downs, getting clues from the "Mad Money" TV show. He asked his stock investment friends how they played the market and which stocks to keep an eye on. He read books and watched several television programs that offered information. In time, he did pretty well, but like any kind of risk, there were wins and losses. One stock he bought did pretty well and made enough money to pay for a new patio. If he found a good stock or a good tip, he would pass it on to anyone who was interested. Some of his co-workers were interested in learning about stocks and he would share with them what he knew, always wanting to help people get ahead. But if the stock went down, he would hear about it from his friends, and because he had given them the tip he would feel so bad about it.

Sandie Gets Sick

Ed was worried about me doing everything, and 2003 was the year from hell. Ed was diagnosed with another bout of cancer and I was having trouble with putting his wheelchair in and out of the car. It seemed to be too heavy and I was getting short of breath. I just thought that I was overtired or something, but one day after having trouble breathing through a song (I sing in the church choir), I came home crying about it and knowing I needed to get to the doctor's the next day. My daughters had done research on the Internet on why I was gaining weight, short of breath, etc., and told me to ask them to check my heart. It was a good thing I asked, because the intern doctor was going to give me an antibiotic and send me home until I mentioned what my daughters had researched. The doctor agreed that some of the symptoms I had were heart-related and yes, she would do an EKG.

They did an EKG and sent me right away to get an echocardiogram. The doctor came out to talk to me and said that I was having cardiac heart failure. My heart was only pumping at 25% and that I needed to be admitted to the hospital for tests and to set up medications. When they did the heart catherization, severe chest pains came suddenly and when I told them, they asked, "1 to 10, how intense?" I said, "How about an 8?" and they put me out. After a couple of days I learned that I had had a heart attack on the table. Statistics say this only happens to one in a thousand when doing this procedure. Later they put me on heart medications and sent me home. They were now concerned about my arrhythmia, so a few months later I ended up having an ICD (pacemaker/defibrillator) put into my chest.

Most upsetting was not being able to go on a trip that Ed and I were scheduled for. We had company-paid airline tickets to Paris for a company event the Friday after I was diagnosed; Ed was to be mentioned as being one of the people that had been with the company the longest, 44 years. Neither of us had ever been overseas before, so it was a big disappointment for us. Ed was devastated with the news of my heart failure and heart attack. He was so used to me being there for him, and it threw him for a loop to see me out of sorts. Our sons flew in to see if they could be of help for a few days.

Our daughter, Tammy, who lives with us and has rheumatoid arthritis, was scheduled to go in for shoulder surgery at the same time all this was happening. My daughter, Denise, who lives near us, had to schedule things to go down to the hospital and be with her while worrying about us. Her husband, Andy, would check every day and do what he could to help us out. Denise, her husband Andy, and my neighbors next door, Harry and Dawn, were my guardian angels and were around most of the time when I needed help. But there were many times when I would have to call for help in the middle of the day when everyone was working or not around.

Ed would have to go to the bathroom but he was getting so weak that he was not able to help get on or off the toilet and he was insistent on using the toilet and not the commode. My strength was limited, so I would look out the door and see if Harry next door or Tom (another guardian angel) across the street, were outside or call one of the neighbors, Ryan or Larry, my son-in-law Andy, my daughter or granddaughters, who were sometimes home during the day, to come help me. Thank God for wonderful people! Sometimes there was no one and I would struggle to get him back in the wheelchair. We did finally get a lift, electric wheelchair and a handicap van to take him places, after my heart attack, so it would be easier on me.

Vacation - August, 2005

Most of our family had planned a trip to go to Lake St. Catherine in Vermont for a week. It was a place where we had brought our children for years when they were young, but not at the same camp. We always loved and enjoyed our time there. So this was a special trip as we hadn't been there for a long time. Ed was not feeling good so I advised the kids that we would not be going, and we decided to take him to the emergency room to find out what was wrong. He was having trouble breathing at times. The doctor there said that he appeared to be having the start of pneumonia. He said, "Here are some pills to take and yes, go and have your vacation, these should take care of it." They gave him another pill to calm him down, but I had told them he couldn't take narcotics, which I think they gave him. He came home and we packed up and got ready to leave with my daughter and her family.

Since he was vomiting some stuff up, I said, "We aren't going!" and he said to just wait awhile; he still wanted to go. The kids did not want to leave us there and Ed still wanted to go, so one of the granddaughters stayed in the van with Poppy while I drove, so she could be there to help him if he needed anything or was getting sick.

So off we went to Vermont. He did well all the way up and we thought that he was going to be good. We stopped at our son's house, since he and his family were going to go with us the next day. We spent the night there, but Ed was still getting sick. He kept saying, "I'll be okay, let's go to Vermont." I was ready to take him back home. We got to the camp and sat him outside while we were all unpacking and he was enjoying the view of the lake. He didn't last long though, and wanted to go lay down. So the boys put him in bed and put the upchuck pan next to him and someone had to be with him all of the time since he was starting all over again. I kept a glass of ice next to him so he wouldn't dehydrate, but it just kept coming up again. He just wasn't doing well. When nighttime came he was getting worse. We decided to take him to Rutland Hospital around 1 am. They did some tests and decided that he had a blocked bowel. He would be operated on the following day.

Unexpected Surgery

He was operated on but things were not improving. After a few days they decided he might have a leak inside and was "going sepsis" (a form of bloodstream poisoning). They would now have to go in again and Ed was not happy. He said that the doctor didn't do it right the first time. He was visibly upset and I could understand, but after talking to the doctors and my doctor back home I understand what can happen when you are operating on the bowel. They advised that if their finger or an instrument just touches the wall it can poke a hole in it. They have to be very careful and they thought they were but something was going on in there. He also had had many bouts of radiation in that area during some of his cancer bouts, so the tissue had become very thin. They kept him in isolation, saying he had MRSA. He was out of the operating room but now he had a hole in his belly called a fistula, where the fesses was oozing out and they had a bag on it. He was not happy. He whispered to me, "No more Italian doctors." We laughed and advised him that nationality had nothing to do with it.

Our family had rented the camp for the week and the grandkids really enjoyed it there. They met another family who had some children about their ages, so that was nice, especially for the teenage girls who met some nice boys and still keep in contact with them. But now it was time for them to go back home.

Ed's sister Rena lived nearby in the small town of Granville, New York, so she offered to put me up until we could get Ed released and back home. We were there six weeks and Ed and I were fighting to get him back home. He would get a little better and they would say okay, he can be transferred to a nursing home. Then he would have another bad day and the insurance company would not pay for an ambulance to transport him to another hospital. So we would hope the next day would be better and so on. This got to the point where I thought I was going to "lose it" and would often break down and cry when his sister and I were together because of the uncertainty of the situation, with Ed not seeming to improve.

One doctor said he could be transferred the next day to a nursing home, so they set it up. The doctor the following day said no, he had to be admitted to a hospital. I would have to pay for the ambulance, since insurance would not pay for it. Ed and I conferred, agreeing that we didn't care at this point, just see what they could do to get us the most reasonable price to transport him to our local hospital back home. It cost us a big bill to move him, but it was worth it just to get him near home again, so my girls and his friends from work could visit with him and I could get some things done at home, too.

My gut feeling before we left for the camp, was that we shouldn't go, but I think that Ed didn't want to let the kids down and he feared that they would cancel their vacation trip. At least, with him being in a hospital up in Vermont, they could go back to the camp and go for a swim and have their vacation. I think he hoped that he might feel better and he always loved being there on the lake. He did get to sit and look at the lake before everything went wrong. We are all glad he was able to do that.

Ed's Last Days

Back home, the doctors were concerned with the MRSA and filling him up with antibiotics. His breathing was getting shallower and he had to be on oxygen more and more. I was getting some kind of cold and not feeling well, but our daughters were stopping by as often as I was, so they told me to stay home for a day or two to get well. We all had to "gown up" to see him.

After he was in the hospital for awhile, he was able to go to the nursing home and use a mobilized wheelchair, which he never wanted. When we would suggest that he get one, he would always say, "I need the regular one for my exercise, I don't ever want one of those things, they make you lazy." He always kept that "move it or lose it" attitude. But now that his muscles were deteriorating, he opted to get one awhile back and had fun in the neighborhood visiting everyone and chit-chatting. We had the same trouble years before, trying to talk him into getting a recliner lift chair so he could stand up more easily and get onto his crutches. One year the kids put their money together and bought him one for Christmas; he loved it after he tried it out.

He was very upset that he had to go to a nursing home. He was only 64 and asked me if I would please work on getting a lift for him to come home. So I bought a lift on eBay that you can install easily and it would help me get him out of the wheelchair and into the bed or bathroom. He couldn't wait to try it out and be home. Working with the nursing center, we opted for him to come home for Christmas because of the lift. He was so excited and kept telling the nurses every day, "I'm going home for Christmas!" So everyone was pepped up for him to return home, especially all of us. Our one son and his family were scheduled to come and everyone was excited. I knew it was going to be a big job for me, but I was willing to try it just to see him come home, even for awhile.

After he came home, it was more than I expected, since

now he had to take a lot more pills. Also, he had diabetes, so that had to be checked four times a day and insulin shots given if required. The lift was working well, and he was so excited that he hoped that he would be able to stay home longer. He would call people and invite them over just to see the lift work.

Christmas 2005

Well, Christmas 2005 was here. We had a lovely Christmas dinner, but he couldn't eat much. He had been saying to us lately, "I'm not hungry!" We sang some Karaoke, which he loved to hear. And the kids would sing to him. We would get him to sing some Sinatra songs for us, if he was up to it. He would have to go lie down a few times during the day.

He looked very pale to me so I asked the visiting nurses to please come to check his blood levels. Well, of course, it was a holiday, and the answer I kept getting was, "He is scheduled for blood work on Thursday." I would say, "I know, but he looks very white to me and I would like them to come sooner." "Well, there is no one that can come sooner," was the answer I got. After a week home, he was having trouble breathing again, yelled for Tammy and me because he was choking. Grabbing the phone, I called 911, while Tammy was holding his head up, trying to help him breathe. The ambulance took him back to the hospital, and needless to say, this time he was staying. His blood levels were very low, and he needed a transfusion. His breathing was labored and he was on a respirator at times. He wasn't doing well. He was not getting enough oxygen.

Tammy was at the hospital one day when one of the respiratory doctors came in and advised him that he had polio syndrome and that his lungs were failing. The only option now was for him to have a tracheotomy. She hated the doctor for being so heartless, as she described it, kind of saying "Well, you have polio syndrome and you are dying." When he heard that, he started saying goodbye to his friends and having long talks with his children and me. I told him that doesn't mean that you are going to die now, it just means your body is giving out little by little and you may have a long time yet, but he just looked at me. He knew what was happening to him.

Polio Returns

After up to 12 or 13 sometimes different chemo and radiation treatments over 24 years, we ended up finding out that his body was giving out, not because of the chemo treatments (although I'm sure they contributed to it), but because his polio had been coming back and slowly taking away each muscle in his body. We both knew it, subconsciously, as we could see that he lost the muscle in his good leg, then his torso, then his arms and hands on one side, now his arm on the other side. We did talk about polio syndrome sometimes, but no one had really diagnosed it until now, so I guess we tried to ignore it.

It probably was for the best that he didn't know everything, since when he heard what it was we could see the look in his eyes and his acceptance as to what was to be. Denise had been staying at the hospital with him and helped to arrange for a conversation with his overseeing doctor. He told him, "I had polio since I was 15 and have battled cancer at least a dozen times for the past 25 years. I've never been a quitter but I know when it's time to let go. I do not want a tracheotomy. It's time." The doctor was very understanding and caring and he told Ed that he understood and respected his decision. He said he would make every effort to see that he was as comfortable as possible. And with that the decision was made.

He took the limited time he had to call his friends and let them know how much he loved them. His buddy Barry, who he rode to work with every day, was at the hospital the day he received the news about the polio syndrome. Barry was visiting his wife, Patty, who was in another hospital room getting some tests done. He stopped to see Ed and was crying before he left. Ed told him how special he was to him and what a great friend he had been over the years, thanking him for all of his help over the years.

All the grandkids sent him their drawings and get well wishes which were hung for him to see. Granddaughters Kasey and Nikki came up with an idea to decorate his room. So they cut, colored and hung lots of fish by strings in the hospital room to make him smile. And later Shannon and Lauren's artwork was added to the décor. My daughters and I would cuddle up with him in bed and go over some of the fun times in our lives. He and his sons had long talks about things they hadn't talked about in years. We would laugh and cry. I would snuggle with him and go over all the wonderful things that we did in our life that we were thankful for and give him lots of kisses. He had to have an oxygen mask on him most of the time now and would take it off whenever he could. He knew that his lungs were giving out and he had limited days. His fight was ending, his struggle was over. Even our efforts to bring back his fight didn't help anymore. He knew the Lord was calling him home.

Ed died on January 10, 2006. He was 65 years old. At the time this book was written, his obituary is still online: http://www.obitsforlife.com/obituary/270696/Sill-Edward.php.

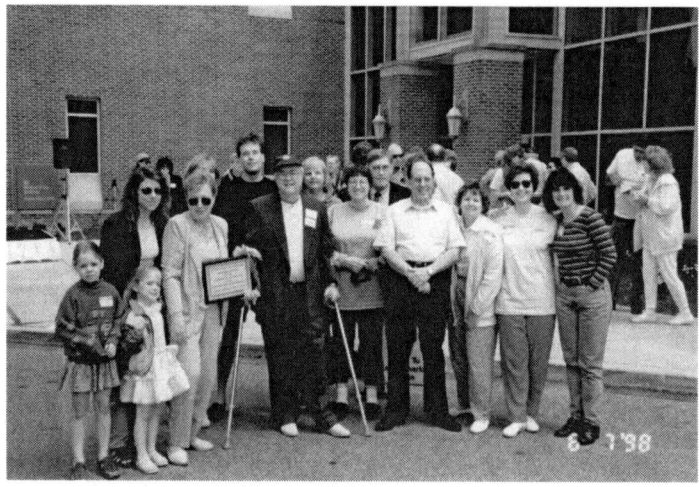

Paoli Hospital presented Ed's office with a plaque for assisting him with his radiation treatments.

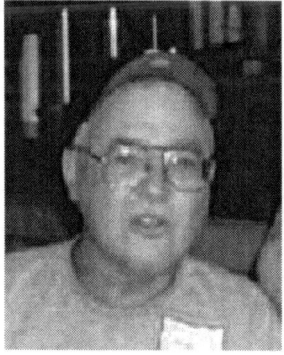

Ed at his high school reunion.

92   *I'm Grrreat!*

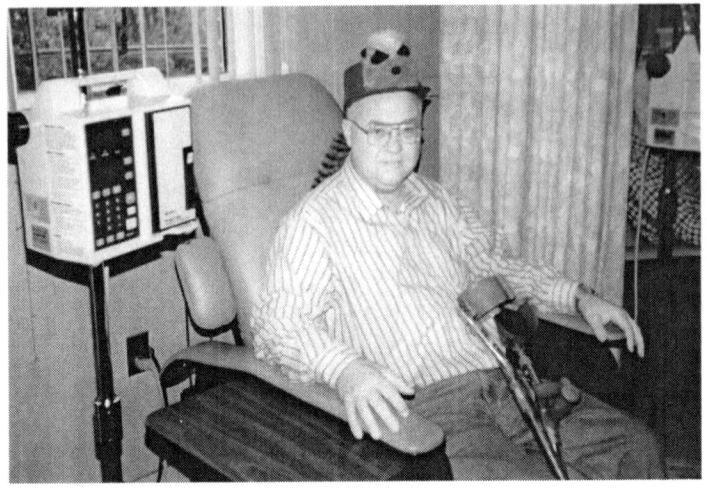

Ed during chemotherapy.

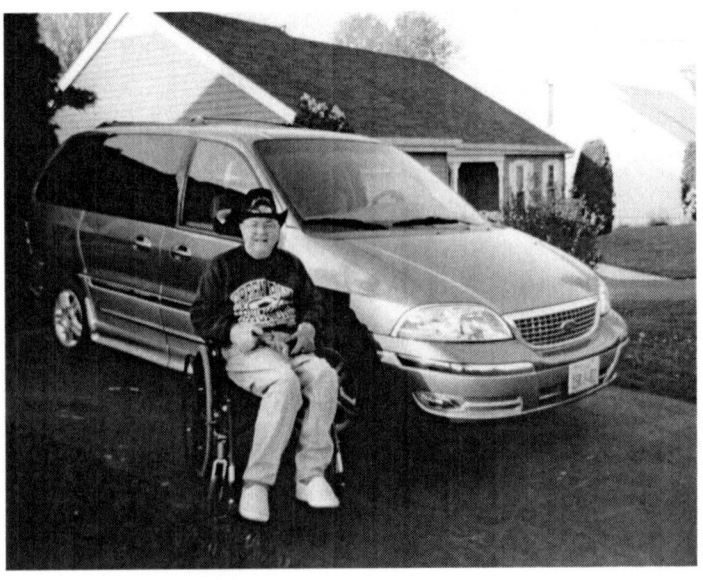

Ed with his new handicapped-accessible van.

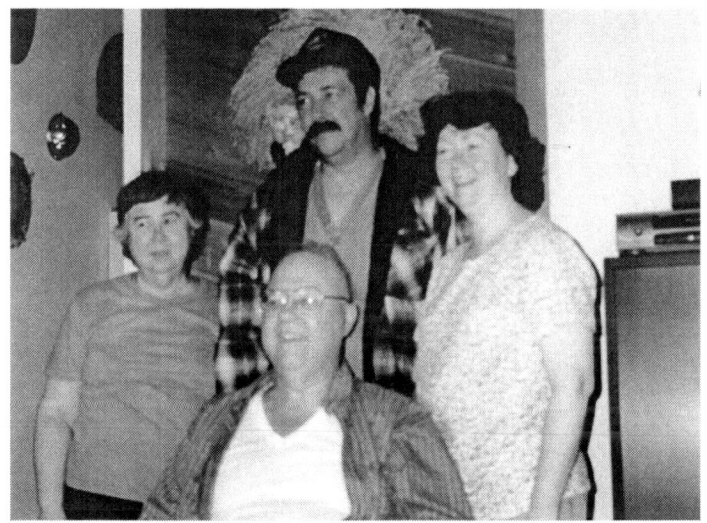

Ed with his siblings, Rena, Feather, and Patty.

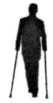

Some Funny Stuff

Shoe Goo

Now Ed had some quirky habits, or "hobbies." Our kids will have to help me here, as I don't know if I can remember them all. Using panel adhesive or "Shoe Goo" for putting things back together was one of them.

For example, he used the panel adhesive to seal the back window of one of the cars we owned as it was leaking. Well, the panel adhesive turned brownish as it aged, cracked and peeled and it was ugly to say the least. People would recognize us by that ugly stuff around the back window. The "Shoe Goo" was used for anything that was broken, not just your shoes, but when the radio had a crack in it. If you just mentioned that something was broken, out came the "Shoe Goo."

His quirkiest "hobby" was trying to insulate our home. One winter we noticed how cold the floors were and he said, "I'm going to fix that." So he proceeded to take some Styrofoam meat packaging out of the trash and wash it. Then he took it and got his shoe-goo or panel adhesive and took the lint out of the dryer filter, put it into the Styrofoam dish and glued it to the ceiling in the basement. Well, I was told to save the Styrofoam and the lint from the dryer for his project and when he had time he would keep doing this to make the floor warmer. Once I said to him, "These are all different colors." He said, "So what? I could always paint over them." I said, "Wouldn't it be easier to just buy some insulation and do this? It would look a lot better." He said, "We can't afford that and why should we, when this works just as well and maybe better." Well, needless to say, we had quite a mosaic-colored ceiling in the basement with yellow, white, pink, and blue Styrofoam dishes. He was quite the innovator and, as you now know, very frugal.

Ed's Nicknames

His friends and family had several different names for him. "Big Ed" was the one most people used. "Big Ed the Pest" was a name he kind of gave himself. This was when he was head of the Babe Ruth League in our area. He would call Ruth Foust, who was the secretary of the league, and say "Hi, this is Big Ed, the Pest!" So she made him a shirt with it printed on the front. The guys in the firehouse nicknamed him, "Sticks," because of the crutches. My kids called him "Harry," after Harry and the Hendersons, which stuck for years. I would tease him and call him "Flapping Lips," because when he was in politics he was always talking to someone or on the phone most of the time.

He would make up nicknames for everyone in the office and the kids had some too. Tammy was "Tammer" or "T," Ron was "Bear" when he was little and "Mouth" when he got older and talked back, Ken was "Clown" 'cause he was always clowning around, Denise was "Neecy" or "Mouse." His friend Ann Marie at work was named "Ketchup". There were several other names at his office, but I can't remember them all. Mark Rozell and Ed gave me the nickname of "Sugarcakes" because I decorated cakes.

Ed the Matchmaker

Ed was quite the matchmaker. He matched several of my friends and his friends together and didn't they get married. One match was his friend, Bob Snyder and a girl Ed worked with named Chris. They got married. Then there was Jola and his friend John. John was about 6'6" and Jola was around 5' or less. I told him no way that was going to work, since she was older than him and he was much taller, but guess what? They got married. Then there was another young girl, Georgia, who I worked with, who he hooked up with an older friend of ours, Hooper, which I thought would go nowhere because of the difference in age, but again they married and are still going strong. I'm telling you, he could have started his own matchmaking business back then.

More of Ed's Hobbies

One of his hobbies was making Popsicle stick dollhouses and

Indian forts. He made several of them, of course the first two were for our daughters and they were so excited as he always included them to help with painting Popsicle sticks or gluing something. The boys helped too, especially when he made the Indian forts. Well, the neighborhood kids wanted to help too and if they helped he would make them one. So he spread the word around the neighborhood to look for Popsicle sticks and bring them to Ed and he would make you a Popsicle fort or dollhouse. Well, needless to say, we had Popsicle sticks coming out of our ears so I would wash them and they would go out on the picnic table and be painted. Ed always made the paint last by watering it down. We had many multicolored ones, as he would always let the kids pick out their colors and they would have to paint the sticks and help with the project.

At work, the guys in his office would have a contest with rubber bands to see if they could pick off the flies that were buzzing around. Ed got very good at it, and he would practice at home too. He could pick one off from quite a ways away. Someone bought him a rubber band gun, which had two places you could place the rubber bands and shoot one after the other. Well, that was the "fun of the week," with everyone trying to see how good they were at shooting flies.

Ed the Fisherman

His biggest hobby was fishing. He taught our kids to fish when they were young. Because the girls and boys would pick on each other, they were taken at separate times. Of course, the boys always thought they were the best fishermen. The girls were another story, they had to have their radio with them and would listen to the music and be singing along with the hook just dangling in the water and a fish would jump on it.

The girls didn't mind catching them, but they didn't want anything to do with taking them off the hook or cleaning them. One of Ed's rules was, if you caught it, you clean it. So he would bring them home and show them how to clean them. The girls were not happy and would tell him they were not going to chop the heads off the fish. They would gag and keep turning their heads. He told them that if you want to fish, you have to learn how to fix them to eat. He loved it and found out that a lot of the kids in our neighborhood had never been. So he made a plan to go every so often and pick certain kids to go with him. Well, you would think that he gave these kids a million dollars. Their eyes would light up and they would be at our door all the time asking if they were going to be picked for the next fishing trip.

During the first few fishing trips, he would have another adult with him, either me or another guy. Sometimes he would go alone and I worried about that, because of his handicap, but the kids always helped him get in and out of the boat with his crutches. He was teaching them how to put the worm on the hook, and how to get the fish off the hook, how to clean them and even how to cook them. He was lucky that no one got badly hooked, as there was always about three or four kids around him and when they swung that pole it was sometimes dangerous. One time at the camp the dog got hooked in the back. Ed made it known that fishing is not just about catching fish but also talking to each other and being together with people you love.

Lunch and Kool-Aid

The kids' only complaint was with some of the concoctions he came up with for lunches. To take all these kids he knew he had to feed them a lunch as they would be on the lake for a few hours and if I wasn't there to help him he made do with what he could find in the house for sandwiches. To make the ketchup stretch he would always add pickle juice to it and sometimes it was a bit much. If it was peanut butter and jelly, at least it wasn't too bad, although my daughter tells me that the jelly would be so thick that it would just squirt out. The other sandwiches were quite a variety of what was leftover in the fridge. The kids now laugh about it. He made Kool-Aid and would mix different kinds together and the kids would guess what the mixture was. But in spite of his love of Kool-Aid, his favorite was orange juice. Most mornings, when we had orange juice, he would drink it down and say "Ah, Nectar of the Gods."

He was like a pied piper in the neighborhood. I used to call our house "The Zoo," because kids and other people were always coming in and out the door. I would answer the door and a kid would be standing there and asking if Ed could come out and play. He had more company, sometimes, than our kids did.

Swimming

Ed loved to swim and he swore that is what helped him to make enough progress to be able to walk again the year I met him. Shortly after he left the rehab, he went to his cousin Marge's summer place where there was a creek that was deep enough to swim in. Swimming daily was his way to gain his muscles back. After we were married, he would go to his sister Rena's pool and swim for hours and sometimes would invite some extra neighborhood kids. (But he would not warn her, so she would be a bit surprised!) We would be invited to go to his cousin Joan's or my sister Jane's pools and, of course, our kids all learned to swim very young. Even our friends who had pools knew he loved it and they would always invite us to their pool on a nice day. The water was very freeing for him and he was able to move his legs and walk like the rest of us.

Neighborhood Baseball

Anyone, child or adult, who walked by was invited up on the porch to chitchat. He helped with the Little League and was President of the Babe Ruth League, as he loved baseball. Our boys were on teams and we were at the fields at least two or three times a week.

He said that he was just getting good with his pitching in his school league when he came down with polio. He was playing football the night he came down with it, and then went home and helped his father dig a foundation for their home in Guilderland.

Anyway, a lot of the kids in the neighborhood were from poor or fatherless families and some of them played in the Little League but didn't always get picked to play. So Ed decided that he would bring them over to a field that was close to our home and play what they call "sand lot ball," when there wasn't a game scheduled or on a Sunday afternoon. They would just pick teams and everyone got to play, good or bad. He would usually pitch or umpire, depending on who was there. He got hit several times with the ball or bat, but he kept on going. He loved seeing those kids able to play ball and have something to do.

Ed the Sports Fan

Ed's favorite baseball team was the Atlanta Braves and for football it was the Green Bay Packers. He had a former coworker and ballplayer friend who now lives up near Chicago. They remained friends with us all of these years, sending him lots of Green Bay items, like a cheesehead and a plaque that reads, "A Green Bay Packer Backer lives here." There was a sign that advised that only Green Bay fans could park here. A neighbor who worked at a billiard place got him a Green Bay ball. He was given a lot of different hats, blankets, coasters, etc. for birthdays and events. There was even a snowman dressed in Green Bay Packer clothes. He loved it. He also loved t-shirts with cute or funny sayings on them. We had to have a Super Bowl party every year, and the last one I remember was with his coworkers. He and his boss, Glenn, (who was a Viking fan) would always go back and forth as to which was the best team, Vikings or Green Bay. They had shirts made and all kinds of trinkets to give to each other to keep the competitiveness going, in a fun way. He had such fun at that party, even though he was going through another treatment at the time.

Ed and his Animal Friends

We had several pets over the years, cats and dogs for the kids. In later years, after those pets passed away, Ed wanted a parakeet. So we had several birds (one at a time, though) -- parakeets, cockatiels, and the last bird we had was a Conure (a small parrot). He was very personable with them. He would take them out and talk to them, teaching them words and making them give him a kiss. Most of them turned out to be pretty smart. The only thing I didn't like was when he brought the bird out of the cage and onto him and the chair because they would poop here and there and guess who had to do clean up? They were messy birds.

The Conure, named "Precious," was very smart but became obsessed with Ed and would start attacking people who came near him, even our granddaughters. We sent "Precious" to a new home when Ed was failing, as he was getting upset with the way he was attacking people and couldn't deal with the loud squawking either. Ed was so good with animals and loved petting all the neighbor's pets. One young neighbor, named Andrea, had a couple of dogs she walked daily through the neighborhood. One of the dogs was "Lindy", and the other "Taylor." She would stop and talk with Ed every time he was out. They would talk about sports, and she would catch him up on what was happening with some of the teams around the area, especially the Phillies.

Dogs would get so excited when they saw Ed that anyone with puppies would put them on his lap and he would take them for a ride in the wheelchair. "Zeke," a beautiful little dachshund who lived down the street, would run like crazy to him when he saw Ed. Across the street at Tom's house, a Pomeranian named Rusty was a puppy when he came to the neighborhood. When Tom saw Ed out in the wheelchair, he would bring Rusty over and put him in his lap. Rusty would get excited for awhile but then would just settle down and lick Ed to pieces. My daughter had two cats and one of them, "Belle," would climb up on his shoulder and wrap herself around his neck when they were at the house. Ed didn't mind, since he was always cold during his last few years.

Memories of Ed

Ed got to know many of the neighbors who walked by when it

was nice out; he was always outside walking or in the wheelchair. He would talk with them about whatever their concerns were, (no wonder our daughter is a counselor), about sports or if they were fighting cancer too, any subject.

My life with Ed was I'm sure different because of his handicap, but it became normal for me. Some of the funny things I remember include the times we were traveling and had to stay at a hotel and try to get him on the toilet there or up on a high bed. There were times when it would be a struggle to get him into the bed and he and I would fall on the floor. We would just laugh and then try again. There were times when he would be frustrated, but most of the time we got through it and laughed about it later.

Ed and I would have been married 45 years in April of 2006. Even though we had ups and downs in our marriage, we always were able to come back to each other and talk about the problems and work them out. We had a comfort zone with each other. Love comes in many ways and I feel that our love grew from all of the trials and wonderful events in our life. I feel an emptiness inside without him but also thank the Lord for all the days he gave us together.

A verse from the Bible reminds me of the way he was. Mt. 9:9-13: Jesus quotes the First Reading and tells the Pharisees and us, "Learn the meaning of the words; I desire mercy (love), not sacrifice." He practiced it by eating with social outcasts, tax collectors, and those regarded as sinners.

Ed greeted all people the same way... he would see a guy

who looked like a hobo walking down the street and say "Hi, how you doing today? Would you like a drink of Kool-Aid?" The kids that I might not have trusted in my home, he would welcome.

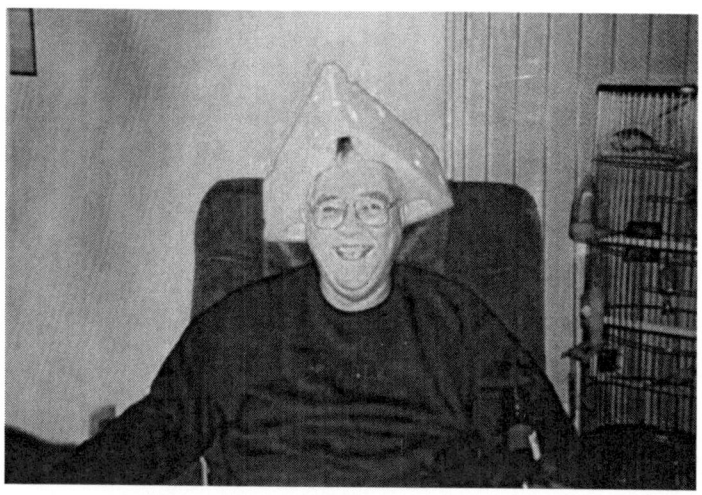

Ed showing support for his beloved Green Bay Packers.

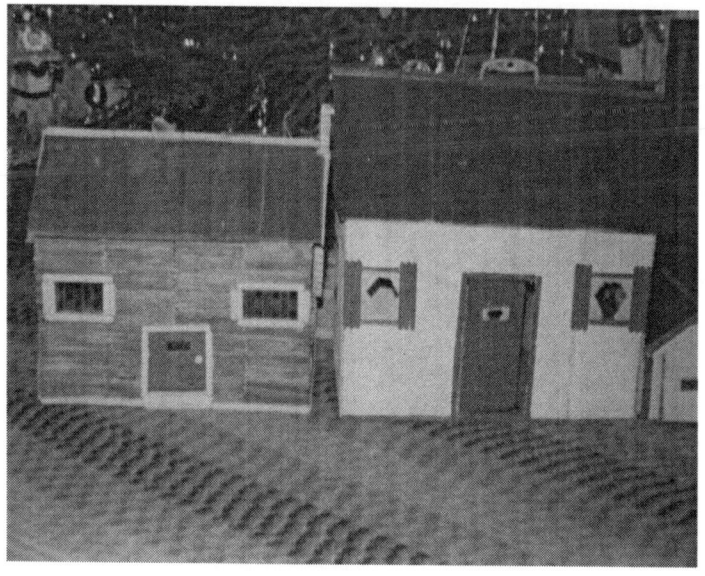

Ed's popsicle stick creations.

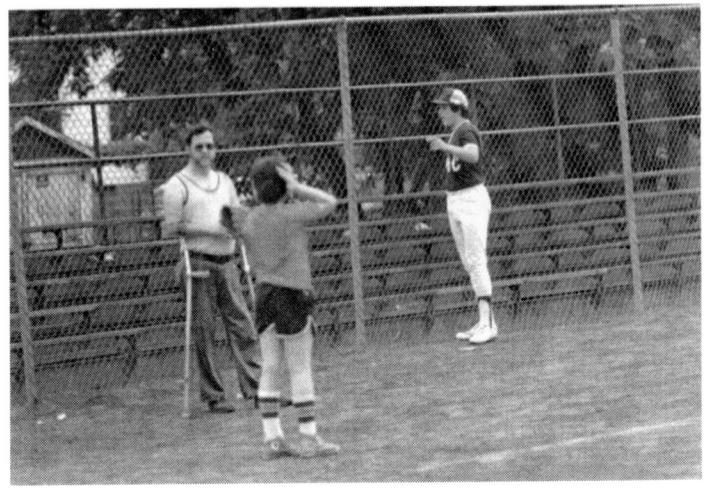

Ed at the Little League ball field.

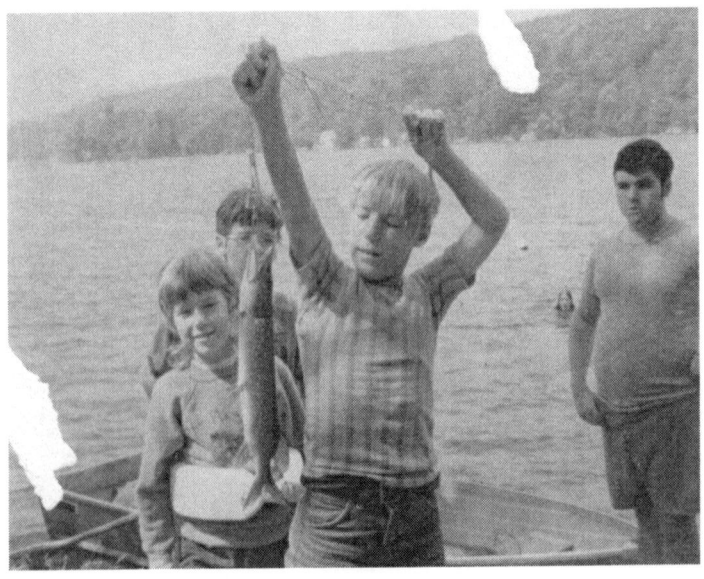

Ed's son, Ken's, big catch.

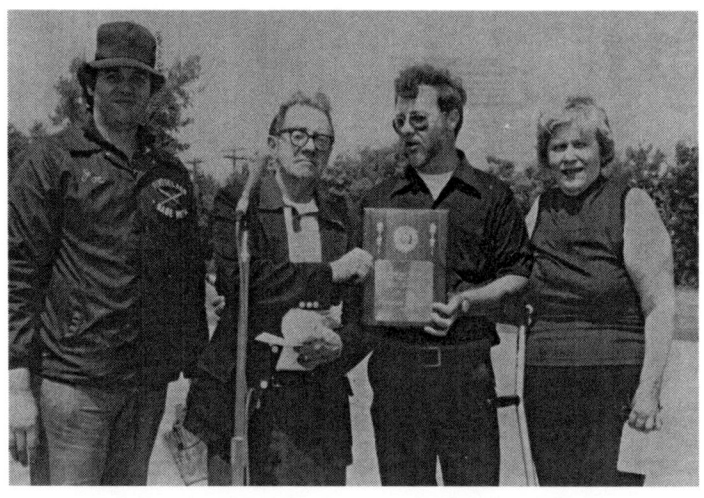

Babe Ruth officers Joe Schepisi, Don Blake, and Ruth Foust presenting Ed with a plaque.

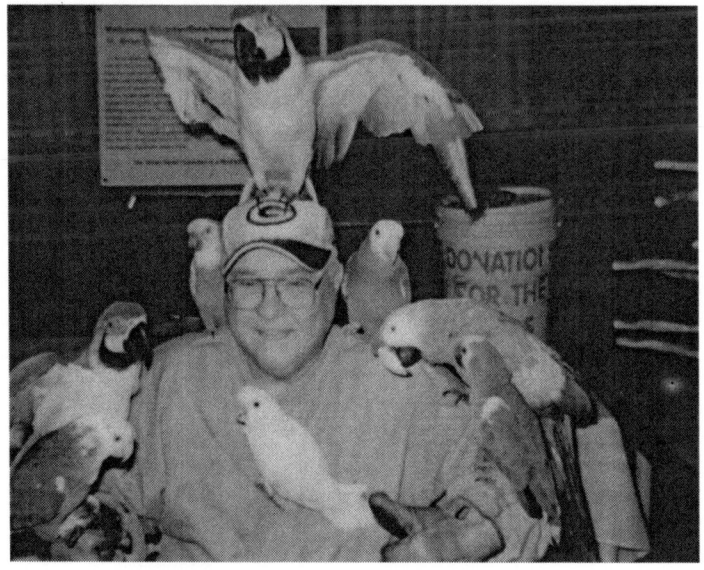

Ed with his feathered friends at a bird show.

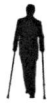

In Their Own Words

ED'S CHILDREN'S LOVE FOR HIM

Tammy

Our daughter, Tammy, wrote this about him when she was younger. (Tammy has suffered from Rheumatoid Arthritis since she was 23 years old. She has some of her dad's immune system problems and struggles daily with the disease.)

"My Dad"
Where do I begin? My Dad, who had to deal with getting a disease called polio at age 16, someone who could no longer chase a dream of playing baseball or football, etc.

But that did not keep him down or stop him from accomplishing other very significant things in his life. He still had fun racing cars, going to drive-in movies with the girls, finishing school and just being a teenager. Then he met Sandra LaMountain who he fell madly in love with. They decided to get married and start a family and that is where I came along, the first child was born and ooh what a lucky girl she was! What I remember most about when I was young, was my dad always wanting to tickle and wrestle with me including arm wrestling. We always had so much fun, he always kissed my cheeks and said "You're the prettiest girl in Rensselaer." Ever since I can remember, he said that to me.

He worked at Sterling Winthrop for years. Everyone loved my Dad, he could sell ice to an Eskimo.

We had many adventures growing up. The thing I loved the most when I was a child was going to camp at Lake St. Catherine every year. Sometimes we would go for a week, maybe two weeks and we would swim and fish, take walks, pick berries, ride horses, and go water skiing. Dad used to get up real early in the morning so we could go fishing. One morning he would take the girls and another morning he would take the boys. As soon as we got back to shore we would jump out of the boat and into the water. We used to love going on the tubes and trying to balance ourselves on them. My mom would call us up to eat lunch and then we'd either sit on the front porch and rock in the rocking chair or go for a walk. We had no TV, only a radio and no phone, it was very peaceful. At night we would go play miniature golf and then go back to camp and start a bonfire and sing or tell stories or roast marshmallows. Then we'd go in and play cards or board games, then off to bed. I loved it there. I never wanted to leave to go back home to get ready for a brand new school year.

I remember many times while I was in grade school, my Dad getting rushed to the hospital or getting sick. Those were sad times for me. I remember crying a lot because I wanted to do something to make him better and I couldn't. He really taught us a lot about compassion and love for people.

Tammy added this later:

> The greatest gift my Dad ever gave me was his TIME.
>
> All through my life growing up, I always remember I could find him either at Coyne Field, fishing, sitting out on the porch, talking to everyone who drove by or walked down our street. He would walk all through the city, but I could always find him and he made time for ME...
>
> He would listen to my latest dilemma and we would problem-solve. It took me years to figure out that my Dad did not take us so we could "catch fish," he took us because he wanted to spend Quality Time with us and that is a gift you cannot buy. Those memories of the time we shared together have brought me comfort (comfort for my blessings) and heartache (heartache for how much I miss him). I was his "T" and he was my Hero...
>
> —Tammy

Ronald

Our son, Ronald, wrote this beautiful eulogy for Ed's services:

> On October 5, 1940, Edward Roger Sill was born. One of four children and brother to Irene, Francis and Patricia, he was full of energy and loved all sports. He was a great young baseball player and played football as well. After a football injury, he came down with polio. He was determined to conquer it and he later began walking with crutches and braces. He met and married Sandra and they raised four children, Tammy, Ronnie, Kenny and Denise. He created a loving family settling in Rensselaer, NY. He became the Secretary and an active member of the local volunteer fire department. He managed and coached men's softball and little league baseball teams as well as being President of the Babe Ruth League. He won the Alderman position in the ward where he lived. During his time as a civil servant, he helped solve many problems for city residents.
>
> He was the pied piper of the neighborhood in Rensselaer where he had the keys to the local ballfield and would turn the lights on at night. He taught baseball and life lessons to any child who came to the park. He loved the Atlanta Braves and was a die-hard Green Bay Packer fan. Another of his famous pastimes was fishing. Ed would say he was a great fisherman, but those that knew him well

would argue that fishing was just another way to spend time with those he loved. He taught many kids to fish who would not have had the opportunity, and in doing so he exposed them to his own, unique and positive perspective on living life to its fullest. A typical weekend around the Sill home included more than a dozen kids ringing the doorbell asking if Ed was going to come out to play or take them fishing.

He was also known in Rensselaer for having an obsession with shoe goo and panel adhesive and found many innovative uses for these compounds.

At age forty, Ed was challenged with lymphoma and given the news that he might have a very short time to live. He simply overcame that battle with cancer and survived approximately a dozen re-occurrences. The health challenges were many, but he never gave up.

Ed and Sandie moved to Pennsylvania for work and he shared his love of baseball with his friends and family. He enjoyed going to games at the Reading Phillies ballfield and really loved attending an occasional major league event. His physical challenges never ceased. Time and time again he came close to death from cancer and each time, by God's will, he rose to the new challenge. Still he had a great attitude and during these times most of you will remember his response to the question, "How are you, Ed?" He would always say, (in his best Tony the Tiger voice), "I'm G-R-R-R-E-A-T!"

Almost every day of his life, Ed would greet his neighbors by walking or wheeling up and down the street. He was loved by those who knew him and as his chapter ended he would be smiling, knowing that these same neighbors honored his passing by placing green and yellow ribbons on some fifty mail boxes where he lived.

God blessed his family and friends with his presence at home this past Christmas (2005) when he took one final victory lap through his neighborhood. We are grateful for having had Ed (on loan) during his short time on earth. As he began the end, he was at peace and with God's grace he was able to pass with dignity, surrounded by his loved ones. If he were here today to give us one last thought, he would simply say, "I did it my way."

Ron also wrote this moving e-mail to his Dad just before he passed:

> 1/8/06
> Dad,
> I have been thinking of you so much and remembering so many hilarious and meaningful times that we had together. It is important to me that you know what an inspiration you have been; to your four children and many of the kids we grew up with in Rensselaer. You have always been my personal hero. Chucky and Grock and Mike Retos and Jeff Benway have all recently told me that

they have never seen a will to live as strong as yours. They also told me that you have inspired each of them and that because of you their lives are better. Benway has totally cleaned up his act and has his own business now. He told me simply "Ed is the toughest man I have ever known" and "they don't make 'em like that anymore." Grock and Retos said the same and Chucky who could easily be my and Ken's adopted brother said it too.

You always liked the Duke (John Wayne) because you said he was tough. I say he could have taken some lessons from the ultimate Duke, Ed Sill. John Wayne didn't beat cancer 12 times, did he? He didn't survive polio and an iron lung and go from lying in bed to dancing with his newlywed wife in a couple of years, did he? I really don't think he ever took 12 kids fishing at once at Kinderhook either, but I could be wrong. I don't think you even know what it is that you gave all of us that makes us think you are great. There is one common thread to the many things you have done for each of us and that you have given all of the kids we grew up with. It starts with love but it is really just time. You gave all of us your time and attention. You have always been patient with all kids and taught and loved us.

We are no longer kids and I have prayed that you will still be here to give us more of your time. I still enjoy talking with you and running things by you to share your wisdom and unique perspective on life and love and work and play. There will never be another Ed Sill, my father, Jared and AJ's grandpa, to take your place. The world will never again be so lucky. However, we each have a piece of you in us that we can keep and hold on to or pass on to our children and them on to theirs. Denise has your wisdom, your eyes, and your cunning to carry her through her challenges in motherhood and her professional decisions. Ken has your patience and sense of humor to help him put life in perspective when times get tough. Tammy has your stubborn determination not to let her body dictate her life and your shrewd money sense to help her make the most out of the least. I have your loyalty and your gift of gab (as mom would call it) and it has and does serve me well as I am never intimidated by a man's position and whether he is a janitor or the president I have learned from you that if he treats me right I will respect him. Jared has many of your traits as well. He and all of your grandchildren have pieces of you that will make them fine men and women.

So you see Dad that although we all must face father time and move on to another chapter, you shall be here with us, forever as we live out our lives. No matter if you are at home watching your 80-inch TV or if you move on to be with our father in heaven. Dad, we can carry the burden if you're tired. We are selfish and want you here with us but we have enough of you inside to guide us if your race has been run.

I just want you to know how proud and thankful I am to be your son. I know that I have been blessed by God to have had you and mom for parents. There is too much I would like to say to write down. I want you to be comforted in the knowledge that we all will take care of the family that you made. Mom and Tam will be fine. We will stick together and continue to love and care for each other as you have taught us.

Remember Dad, what you taught me before Randy Travis sang about it; "it's not what you take when you leave this world behind you, but what you leave behind you when you go." Say hi to Mark Rozell, Al Pal, Uncle Gary, Grandma Sill and Gram LaMountain and all those we love who have run before us. I love you, Dad.

—Ron

Kenneth

Our son, Kenneth wrote this beautiful essay for a college project about the family:

Family Legacy Essay, April 3, 2008

How is it that the soft vibrations caused by the movement of the strings of a bow on a violin, resonate so loudly when they bounce off of the human soul? Sometimes we see the waves coming at us, as we are captivated by watching the symphony orchestra.

Other times, they sneak up on you and you don't even know why, but your physiology starts to change. Whether the background music in an epic movie, or the accompaniment in a popular song, their power is difficult to escape. The ripple effect they cause is analogous to pebbles dropped into the water on one side of the lake while a wave is felt on the other side. It is hard to explain, but somehow there is a connection between these seemingly disparate events.

The experiences we have in our lives, whether spiritual or physical, have the same power as the strings on the bow or the pebbles. Initially they may seem small or possibly insignificant, but later in life you come to understand and appreciate the power and significance they truly possess.

Thus begins my story about a young boy growing up in a small city in upstate NY. It is a cool, crisp, sunny fall morning and Sunday Mass has just ended. Songs of the morning service still echo loudly in my head as we climb into the family car and head for home. Mom would get up early on Sunday mornings to get my brother, my two sisters and I polished up and ready for Sunday service. Having to manage four children, a husband with polio, a dog and a cat..., mom found solace and rejuvenation in the Church.

Although it took some prodding and a great deal of "shhs" to get us to the church, not to mention maintaining order while we were there..., we eventually grew to appreciate mom's spiritual connection.

Some of fondest memories came from the journey home Sundays after church. When I grew older, my mom allowed my siblings and I to walk home from church. Having our cup completely filled with a week's worth of religious spirituality, we ventured on our fabulous ten-minute journey home. The spirituality that I found in church was simply a small piece of the overall spirituality I would gain on a Sunday morning. It was on the way home that I got a Ralph Waldo Emerson-like appreciation for the simple things in life. Although I must admit, at times it felt more like an Indiana Jones archeological adventure! My weekly journey would lead me over two hills, across railroad tracks, past a creek, through a field and across a street.

Time seemed to stand still as a child in the late 1960s and early 1970s. My journey homeward would involve frequent stops to smell the flowers along the creek, the frequent jaunts to catch a butterfly or grasshopper, and the improvement of my pitching skills as I would toss rocks at any piece of debris that may have found its way into the creek. Like a fish to a shiny lure, I would notice something floating in the creek, or a piece of pottery stuck in the dirt, and I was hooked. These attractions provided me a forum to practice my archeological skills as I would immediately work toward dislodging these artifacts from whatever was clutching them. Much to my chagrin, the treasures that I would uncover consisted mainly of broken bottles probably left behind by past adventurers, such as I treasure less, (other than some occasional loose change found in the road) I would venture onward until I reached my destination.

When I was not attending church, or becoming one with nature, I focused a great deal of my energy on playing sports. My dad provided the fuel for what became one of my greatest passions. I would later learn from my grandmother that my dad was a great baseball player until he was stricken with polio at the age of sixteen and that he loved the game as well. His passion for the game may have been slightly curtailed by the polio, but it never slowed him down. He was the consummate optimist. As a matter of fact, I am pretty sure if you were to look up optimist in the dictionary, low-and-behold you would see his picture jump off the page. His optimism was contagious in general, but even more so when it came to teaching others what he knew about the game of baseball.

Dad would spend hours with my brother and me tossing the baseball in the street or on the local ball field. He introduced me to the game at a very young age, as I started playing baseball around the age of three. Dad coached many teams from Little League and Babe Ruth to fast-pitch men's softball. Dad's guidance and instruction was provided with the following recipe: a heavy dose of toughness, a great deal of discipline, and a whole lot of fun. Growing up in the pre-Nintendo generation, virtual sports were not part of my game playing experiences. The bulk of my day was spent playing games that provided real world experiences.

Playing both pickup games and organized sports, (primarily football, baseball and basketball) I learned many things. Not the least of which was teamwork, leadership, and commitment. All of these team sports help to develop a greater sense of teamwork. In order to be effective and win, the team must work cohesively toward achieving their goals. Even though these sports are team-based, they still require leadership to achieve their goals.

The leadership qualities I obtained were gained primarily from my role in baseball performing the duties of pitcher. Generally considered the leader on the baseball diamond, the pitcher is the person who has a great deal of control over the outcome of the game. The measure of an effective leader is seen in his ability to motivate others towards the accomplishment of a goal. The teams that I pitched for won many titles and trophies. The achievement of these accolades could only be realized by hard work, determination and commitment. Commitment was learned by arriving to the field on time, staying later than everyone else to practice a new pitch, or practicing until late into the night under the street lights. The invaluable lessons my dad provided, by teaching me the virtues of teamwork, leadership and commitment, have become the bedrock for my success in business.

As I look back now, I see how these relatively insignificant-at-the-time experiences and interactions have now become the foundation for who I am. The legacy that my family provided me, form the foundations for who I am and what I believe in.

It is said that it takes a lot of little things to make up one big thing. Like the strings on the bow of the violin, or the pebbles dropped into the lake, something that seemed insignificant at the time, now has great significance.

Denise

Our youngest daughter, Denise, who was the last to talk to him before he went into a comatose sleep, writes this:

"Well Mouse, there's only two people in this world that have it all figured out – and I'm not so sure about you anymore…"

That was the essence of the #1 greatest man in my life, my father, Edward (Harry) Sill.

My earliest memory is one of being scooted up the stairs as a toddler and hanging onto him as he worked his way to the second story of our home on his backside – one step at a time. As a byproduct of having polio as a kid, he couldn't walk up stairs like most people. With my brothers and sister carrying his crutches to the top, he would set me down, roll over onto his hands and knees, walk his hands up the wall; grab the crutches and joke with us until we all piled into someone's bed for story time.

There were "good nights" and "I love yous" shouted into the darkness until all our names were used. Sometimes we also went down The Walton family names until we got to "John Boy" and laughed at our familial wit. I remember a childhood that was safe and nurturing, loving and disciplined, filled with laughs and screaming matches; but mostly honest about feelings and the realities of life (both the joys and the sadness).

Every year, there were traditions like snuggling up around him and mom on the couch for The Wizard of Oz and Willy Wonka and the Chocolate Factory. At Christmas time, we couldn't wait for Rudolph, the Grinch, Santa Claus is coming to town, Snow Queen, and Frosty The Snowman. We were together.

In spring and summer all four of us looked forward to our weekend "fishing" trips. We'd help dad make and pack lunches of sandwiches and Kool-Aid and have all our friends ready to load up a couple of cars for Kinderhook Lake and "strawberry bass." Tammy and I did the worm, hook and guts thing in our early years but later cared more about tanning and the radio. It didn't matter why, but we looked forward to it and could always count on it.

We swam! Whether it was at a lake or in Aunt Rena or Aunt Joanie's pool, we were all taught how to swim. For dad, swimming was total freedom. There was no struggle or restriction from his disability. All four of us fell in love with swimming.

There were daily traditions too. We ate dinner together each night as a family – no matter what! This was probably my father's most stringent rule! I remember cringing if the phone rang during dinnertime or even worse, if the doorbell rang. Dad would get up from his chair and quite angrily inform the caller or visitor that they were never to interrupt our family mealtime again!

My father was frugal with money spent on "things." We did not have a big house or expensive clothing, furniture or cars. However, he did have his priorities. He and mom made sure that our family vacation at Lake St. Catherine in Vermont was planned every year. There was more fishing, swimming, game playing and snuggling (this time by the campfire). While there, it seemed as though we were the richest family in the world! Later, I would come to understand, we were.

When we became teenagers, I think he was sad. Mom worked long hours by then and they had their challenges both in their relationship and careers as well as managing four adolescents who were all going in different directions. Being the youngest was, to me, both a blessing and a curse! Some of my most special moments with him occurred during this time; though some very painful memories as well. We walked. Because of his polio, dad's life mantra became one of "move it or lose it." He knew from a young age that he had to keep exercising to keep his strength, so we walked. We walked around the neighborhood and at the ball field, by the riverfront and at every outside event. I loved being with him. I loved talking with him. I loved listening to his thoughts about life. He told me not to ever let anyone treat me badly. He told me I could quit my year and a half-long job at Burger King because I was unhappy and being mistreated. He told me how smart I was. He told me it would be OK.

Then my father got cancer. I think I was about 18 or 19. Ron and Tammy came home from different parts of the country. We were all together again! For a moment in the hospital room we were that young strong family and I felt him gathering his strength.

He would be challenged many more times with the cancer and each time it came, he drew his strength from the presence and love of his family. One could see and feel the energy shift when he had us all together. He was quite proud and amused when we all paraded into his hospital room with his "unique" collection of zany hats displayed proudly on our heads!

He had "the talk" with me that changed everything during his last battle with cancer. He was lying in his bed one night and I jumped in with him like we all still did on occasion, and he said "Mouse, I'm ready to go soon, I've lived a great life, I have the greatest family in the world. I got to see my grandchildren..." And through my tears I said "Dad, I'm not ready, we can't lose you... please Dad," and I talked about Mom, Tam, Ron, and Ken and how they would be angry and wouldn't let him quit and how much we still needed him. I told him it would be OK. After that talk, I called my brothers and told them to come because dad needed their strength and they both came and gave it to him, by then, in the hospital room. He gathered his strength and won another battle!

My dad died January 10, 2006 from the effects of polio, which, we now know, typically occur later in life. He felt his body changing rapidly despite his daily exercise and amazing love for life and family. None of us really understood this post-polio syndrome. We never understood our father to be disabled! We had the cancer thing figured out but this was a snake we thought he had conquered long ago. As confused as we all were, his doctors were even less aware, which created a much greater challenge as we fought this invisible war.

When he knew he would not live without the assistance of a trachea, he decided to take back some control and talked with the doctor about a plan for dying with dignity. I spent those moments trying to be for him what he had always been to me. I was so sad and so scared. This was a walk we had never been on and neither of us wanted to take; but I loved being with him. I loved talking with him. I loved listening to his thoughts about life. I knew what my job was because he taught me long ago; so I didn't let anyone treat him badly. I knew he could quit because he was unhappy. I told him how smart he was. I told him it would be OK.

Denise said the following words at Thanksgiving 2008, the first time we were all together again since saying goodbye to him!

"It's good that we are all able to be together as a family and with friends to celebrate our connection with each other—and give thanks.

"It's sometimes hard to know how to show gratitude in the midst of loss and it's even harder to know how to express the contradicting feelings of grief and joy that I think we are all feeling at being together without you, (our father/husband).

"I think it was important for us to be apart since you left Dad, because I believe we all had some business to take care of. We needed to come to terms with our own feelings and explore the meaning of our lives without you in them before we could begin to do what you would want and expect from us; which is for us to continue to function as the close, loving, supportive family you and Mom created.

We know that our work now is to forever try to honor you in our healing and, as we assess our personal and family choices, make every effort to raise the next generation of Sills with the integrity, courage, strength and togetherness you modeled for us throughout your life."

GRANDCHILDREN'S REMEMBRANCES

Shannon and Lauren

Our granddaughters, who were 4 and 5 at the time Ed died. They are the daughters of our son, Kenneth, and his wife, Kelly.

Lauren and I wanted to say he always sang old McDonald to us on the phone. I also remember Poppy mispronouncing (our dog) Natey's name a lot. We love him and miss him. And have his Popsicle stick house to remember him.

Nicole Taylor

Our granddaughter, Denise's daughter.

Dear Poppy,
I miss you every day. We all do, but sometimes things are easier because we know you're still with us. I hope you're happy wherever you are.
There are so many things I wish I could ask you about.

So many times I've wanted to call you for advice. I'd give anything to hear your voice again, asking "Where's my kiss?" or "Hey Snick, can you take off my shoes for me?" I promise I wouldn't fight with you about it. I'd leap to do it.

I wish I could hold your hand, or push your wheelchair down the sidewalk—as a woman. I wish you could see me as I am now, instead of knowing me as that ungrateful, selfish little girl. I'm strong now. I'm different. I'm not afraid to talk to people anymore, I'm not afraid to help a stranger, or really listen to someone when they speak. I know it seems like I never listened to you, but everything you taught me to be is a goal I work towards every day.

Sometimes I try to replay our conversations in my head, even though it was so long ago, and there were too many to count. There are too many to recall in one sitting. I see the comics in the paper sometimes and I think of you. I think about how we used to read them together. I think about how I never really knew anything about you until you were gone. I wish that I had shown you how much I loved you. I wish you had finished telling me your life story.

Every time I see the tree in the front yard, and the old chairs waiting on the porch, I think of you. I see you for a moment, smiling at me. Sometimes I feel like we're playing ball, and you're throwing me a ball of life and saying, "Catch."

I'm sure you know this, but you have a great

granddaughter now, her name is Bailee. I hope we can all teach her the things you've taught us. I hope that I don't let you down anymore.

It's been years since you've been gone, but I carry you in my heart always.

Love, Nikki

"This one time, when I got my first boyfriend, Poppy said, "I thought I was your boyfriend!" He sounded so funny and hurt, I'll never forget it. You will always be in my heart and thoughts. Love,"

—Nikki (granddaughter)

Kassandra Taylor

Our granddaughter; Denise's daughter.

My Poppy has influenced me for the rest of my life. I spent, what I thought was a great deal of time, with my Poppy when I was younger, now I wish I would have never left him for even a minute. I am my Poppy's granddaughter 110%. I go out of my way to talk to strangers daily, I pick up litter when I see it along the sidewalk, and most importantly, I love my family. We took many walks, it gave us a chance to talk, and get to know each other. Those walks we shared would involve stopping and talking to everyone we saw, whether we knew them or not. My Poppy could make conversation with anyone and put a smile on the most miserable person's face. I envied the way he did that, and studied it thoroughly. When we saw garbage on our way he would either have me pick it up or he would get it himself using a grabber. Being wheelchair-bound was no inconvenience for him.

My Poppy taught me how to paint. Guiding me in the right direction and correcting me gently, we must have painted all of the trim in the house. He used rubber bands instead of fly swatters to kill flies in the house. (That's still something I just cannot seem to get down.) My Poppy always had a jar of pickles, one that we had to raid every time we were over! Karaoke turned into a family tradition, anything involving family became tradition. Cards became another family event; he taught me how to play pinochle with the best of them. He was always patient, everything I did was perfect for him as long as I had tried my best and asked for help when I needed it. When I needed an answer, he had it and taught me how to find it for myself, and when I was scared he was my protector. Who knew a grandfather could be so many things? I am resentful that he is gone; I really could have used his advice a few times since then. I am sad because my daughter will never get to meet him, but in the words of my Uncle Ron, (his son) "The good news is, there is a little bit of him in all of us." He is with all of us in our own ways and memories.

Every time I go out of my way to say, "Hi" to someone

who seems to be having a bad day, or make conversation with someone who is alone waiting for the bus, I feel him, smiling, because he'd be doing the same thing. I hope that he is proud of the woman I have become, because I would not be who I was without his contribution. I can only wish that everyone is so lucky to have someone like him in their lives, but I know that cannot be. I was the luckiest girl in the world to have Edward R. Sill as my grandfather, and there really is no one out there like him. I love and miss him so much, words really cannot describe it.

—Kasey

"You always were "my favorite Poppy!" There was no one like you ever and I loved painting and fishing with you! I will never sell or get rid of those Popsicle houses you created. I remember helping make them and really feeling like I had accomplished something. You were my best friend, I told you everything. I love you!"

—Kasey

Aaron Sill

Our grandson; Ronald's son.

Poppy was an awesome grandpa; I remember going for walks with him and we'd talk the whole time about random things. I loved being around him, he was so nice and friendly and cared for everybody more than himself. I loved him very much and I'll always miss him.

Kristopher Sill

Our grandson; Kenneth's son.

"The Man Who Loved Life"

My grandfather was a loving sentimental man who loved me as well as the rest of the family with all he had. He always knew how to make me smile and bring warmth to my heart every time I would give him a great big hug.

In my early childhood days I remember Gram would go out and buy us two boxes of Popsicles; Pop and I would sit there all day and eat every last one of the Popsicles just leaving the sticks behind. Each Popsicle stick we would collect went into a jar until we had enough to build an Indian fort and play Indians and cowboys.

I can still remember those endless karaoke nights with you and the rest of the crazy Sill family, those days when we would shoot everything in sight with our rubber band guns, and then sit on the couch watching your Packers play, while you had your cheesehead on routing for them from beginning to end.

We would always find a way to have fun. I can still remember those cool summer days when we would go fishing. Pop and dad would always compete for who could catch the bigger fish. I later joined the competition when I got older. Sometimes we would end the day great and others empty-handed, but we always had a blast enjoying each other's company. I can't remember a moment that was ever dull (although he was a little hard on me from time to time, it was for my own good) with the man who has truly inspired me to be who I am today my Poppy, Ed Sill.

The memory of you will live on forever in my heart, and the rest of the Sill family. I miss you and love you with all my heart. I know you're watching over us from heaven. You are gone, but will never be forgotten. You fought for your life every day I will fight to keep the memory of you alive forever... Edward Roger Sill, 10/5/40 – 01/10/06.

—Kristopher

Jared Sill

Our grandson; Ronald's son.

Edward Roger Sill was not just a friendly neighbor, loving father, and Packers enthusiast. "Poppy," though on a small scale in the grand scheme of the things of the world, made an impact on the lives of a considerable amount of people. I like to think of Poppy's life as a chain reaction: the start of an incredibly proud tradition that is the Sill name. Poppy was and is the anchor who kept the lives of his family from spinning out of control. I personally share not only a deep love for my grandfather, but also a deep, unmatched respect for the man who lived his life in a way that not every man can do. No mountain was too large for Poppy. He has set the bar high for his children, grandchildren, and great-grandchildren alike. To me, the small things he did were the most important. Rides to the gas station for candy, or "shooting" the Indians on western movies together were so meaningful. In all honesty I could go on for a long time about ways he has touched my life as well as others.

Finally, through all the physical suffering I witnessed him endure, my very last visit with him summed up him as a person. Through his last sickness, laying on a hospital bed, in pain, he wore an enormous smile, clear blue eyes a-glowing, with a ham and cheese sub that Dad and I snuck in for him. I love you Poppy, and I thank you for everything you did. Though our time together was shorter than I would have liked, I appreciate every moment we shared. I hope you and the Lord work together to mold me into the young adult I am becoming, and I pray I will be half the man you were.

—Jared Sill

Edward Sill

Ed's namesake, his nephew.

"My first memory of my Uncle Ed"

I'm pretty sure my first memory of Uncle Ed was in the mid-80s. He was up visiting Grandma and was going to come see us too. I was told he was who I was named after, which at the time didn't seem to mean much, but even then, it seemed special to me somehow. It had me curious anyway, for I was in the front yard waiting expectantly.

He drove into the driveway slowly, with a smile when he looked at me. He knew me and called me by name, though I had no previous memory of meeting him. I watched him get out of his car, (I think it may have been his Camaro) and immediately it became apparent that he wasn't "normal" in the sense that he used two long gray metal things to pull himself up and walk with. He had an almost jerky way of moving his legs when he walked. It seemed funny and alarming for it was the first time I encountered him.

However, he had no problem lifting me up with a big smile on his face while saying how big I'd gotten. And I remember him surprising me with a matchbox car, red, which he somehow had pulled out of nowhere. How did he know I liked to play with cars? I made roads in dirt and bridges and other extravagant obstacles. It was one of my favorite things to do. Also, he said my name like a professional, with ease. I remember him later lifting me up into his lap and just questioned me on my siblings, and toys, and activities, and anything else that had to do with me, making me seem unique. From that first meeting I knew I was somehow special to him and him to me.

So I associated my uncle with blue Camaros, gifts that either catered to my interests or started new ones such as coins, and crutches. When I broke my ankle during the spring of '92 and spent the summer on crutches, it was no big deal, my uncle used them, and so could I.

My current interests still remain cars, and design. I am Ed, named after my uncle. No matter what life throws at me, I think of someone who had it worse, but could lift me up like a feather, although he looked like he couldn't lift anything. Every time I think of him, I see a special huge smile just for me, and I see someone extraordinary. I'm proud to have been named after him. He gives me strength to this day if I ever feel down.

Love, Eddie

ED'S SIBLINGS

Irene (Rena) Sill DeMeur

Ed's older sister.

"My brother Ed"

Days when I felt lonely or depressed, the phone would ring and that wonderful voice would say, "This is "Big Ed," turning my mood around. He always seemed to know when I needed his support and was always there for the whole family. People liked him. Ed could make friends with just about anybody and those friendships lasted a lifetime. I remember how bravely he faced his numerous illnesses and refused to admit defeat. His sense of humor always carried on. How much I miss that voice, intelligence and spirit and always will. I miss you Ed.

Your sister, Rena

Frances (Feather) Sill

Ed's younger brother (by 15 years).

Hi, I'm "Feather," Ed Sill's younger brother. This was the nickname that "Big Ed" tagged me with for my entire life. It doesn't hurt—not at all.

Ed always had time for me and every person who he touched with his life force.

He influenced every person in a positive way, at church, ball games... Every weekend loading up his Olds or Chevy with as many children he could pack in to go fishing.

He'd pitch a ballgame for the kids, making sure everyone had a good hit, no a great hit and feeling like a star, and he was there to make sure this child would glow in "Big Ed's" life force.

"Big Ed" will watch over each and every person that he

touched. He'll watch from Heaven with his dog, Spunky. I'll see you, whenever that is Ed, so leave a couple of big ones in the fishing hole for me when I get there. Like Jesus was a fisher of men, "Sticks" was also a good fisher of men.

Love you Always,

Francis C. Sill "Da Fed"

Patricia Sill LaValley

Ed's youngest sister and his brother-in-law John.

(John) "Ed, whenever I felt down and depressed, I would tell Pat I need an "Eddie Fix." A trip to PA would always perk us up. You and your aura would make things better. We will miss those trips. You always gave us support. It was hard moving west and being so far away, but the phone calls were always great. I know you were happy for us. Will always miss you and love you."

(Pat) He was so wonderful to all of us and to the animals. I remember him with the dogs, cats, birds and even the horses. I remember everyone laughing at the time you admired our new horse, who turned out to be a wild deer that jumped the fences to get in with them.

Eddie laughed all the time with us. I remember his ability to treat everyone the same until they proved they weren't worthy of his trust. He loved children and taking them fishing. I remember him coming up to the house with one of his neighborhood kids and swimming in the hot tub. I recall how much he loved the swimming pools at our house, and Joan's. He told me it was the only time he could move so freely because of the polio damaging all of his leg muscles. He always treated his Mom with great respect and love, and unlike some of us he never yelled at her. He was the kind of man who could make friends with men and then treat us kids great too. Overall I felt he was the best big brother a sister could ever have.

John admired him a great deal because he made being related more like he was a brother not brother in law. Like the karaoke music nights with Eddie, singing Elvis and John, doing Tiny Tim. What a hoot! John says he never laughed so much and so hard in his life. We used to love how Dino would sit on his shoulder at breakfast He loved showing everyone around PA and made a great tour guide. He loved sharing his friends with us, and having dinner with everyone. He loved speeding down the ramps at the restaurants in his wheel chair. He made John a "wreck" one night, thinking he was going to crash since he was going so fast. John really enjoyed pushing him around in his wheelchair when we were touring around to see things. It was a great pleasure and honor to do that for him. He was pretty special to all of us, and we will remember him forever.

Love, John & Pat

ED'S CLOSE FRIENDS

Art Haughton

This is from one of his best friends, Art (who passed away from cancer in October, 2008). Artie was a foster child who Ed's cousin had cared for, and he would stay over at Ed's house a lot. They became good buddies.

Ed was more then my best friend, and a great person, to me he was like a brother. It's hard to put into words; a lifetime of great memories. I believe God knew he was a special person. By choosing the first two numbers in the date 1/10/2006, Eddy went to heaven, One and Ten. One—Eddy will always be in our memories as a great friend and a One of a Kind person. Ed was a "Ten" in the way he lived his life, with his family and friends always helping in any way they could. Those two numbers together make One Hundred and Ten, the percentage he gave to everything he did.

Everyone has their special memories of Ed, during both the good and the hard times. And the challenges that faced him throughout his life with polio and cancer. By never giving up and fighting for his life, that made him a hero in many ways. By always keeping a positive attitude and a great personality. No matter how bad a situation was, he would make a bad day into a good day, with the thought that tomorrow will be a better day. Eddy enjoyed his friends and family and lived his life to the fullest, in every way he could. I feel good and proud, that we were always good friends, and we hung around together from our teens until now, and shared some good times. These memories will never be forgotten and will always be part of my life.

—One of Eddy's best friends, Art

Glenn Steinke

Glenn was Ed's last boss, someone he had a great relationship with and of course there was a "competitive edge..."

A Rememberance: "Big Ed" Sill—Brother, Mentor, and Partner-In-Crime

By Glenn Steinke

I'm not sure exactly why Ed Sill was tagged with the nickname "Big Ed". It could have been his larger than life optimism. It could have been his vast product knowledge of Sterling Winthrop Pharmaceutical development compounds. Or maybe the big laughs he would create with a joke or funny story or a smile. Wherever and whenever the nickname began, he was always "Big Ed" to me.

"Big Ed" Sill and I became fast friends when we met at Sterling Winthrop in the summer of 1993. We shared a lot of laughs as troublemakers and became very close friends, especially during his chemotherapy regimen at Paoli Hospital. In summary, Ed was a big brother, a friend and a mentor. His love and pride of his work accomplishments was only trumped by his love of his wife and family. (And also perhaps trumped by his love of the Green Bay Packers.)

"Trumped" took on a new meaning for me when Ed taught our entire department at work to play pinochle during lunch breaks. We would sometimes have two or three games going on at one time. When the weather was nice, Big Ed would grab a Frisbee and encourage us to play outside. If you ask anyone, Ed seemed to never have a bad day. He responded with a hearty "grrreat!" when asked how he was doing no matter the hour.

You could make a strong and solid argument that Ed was dealt a bad hand from a health perspective. His reduced mobility was apparently due to being out of school on a particular day in his youth—missing the polio vaccine. From his accounts, Ed was diagnosed with cancer in his early 40s. He was repeatedly counseled when the cancer re-appeared in the short month durations he had left to live.

Listening to Ed recall these events, they seemed more like stories than facts. They were communicated as if they were minor speed bumps that would not derail Ed from his positive outlook—no matter the gravity of the diagnosis. "Big Ed" beat the odds in so many ways and proved the experts wrong.

Ed was passionate about his many contributions at Sterling Winthrop and later Sanofi—which helped to bring new medicines, therapies and new optimism for patients-in-need. During an FDA inspection, Ed once took the lead and impressed the young lead auditor with his product knowledge and his depth of understanding. He was always willing to share all his knowledge and never selfishly keep it for his own job security. He was a teacher to all who wanted to learn more about his encyclopedic knowledge and experience.

But these facts are only footnotes in the memories I carry from our friendship. Big Ed loved life and made me laugh. He made me think about the power of positive thinking and how the odds could be consistently overcome. He taught me how to invest in the stock market, properly cast a reel off a fishing boat, play practical jokes on annoying coworkers and he always made me forget he had any limitations or worries or bitterness about the cards he was dealt. Ed played his hand no matter the circumstance and won the admiration of myself and others every time.

It may be coincidence (but still interesting to note) that my son Noah is now a tremendously passionate Green Bay Packers fan. Just like "Big Ed" Sill. This is especially troubling to me, actually—as a lifelong Minnesota Vikings fan. Yet in reality, it's only more proof that Ed's presence is somewhere near—pulling strings to both torment me in fun and remind me that he's not forgotten. Still a troublemaker.

And if I had to guess now, I would offer that the "big" in Ed's nickname is the significant influence he continues to have on my daily life. I'm sure he's laughing somewhere from a distance as my son puts on his Packers jersey, cheesehead hat and fearless attitude every football Sunday.

Big Ed? Are you listening? I'll get you for this!

Doctor Fox

A very special letter from Ed's cancer doctor, Dr. Stephen C. Fox:

> Dear Mrs. Sill & Family,
>
> I want to express my condolences on the passing of Ed. How to do this with someone of his character that I have known for two decades is another story, but I do need to try.
>
> From the onset, Ed impressed me as an individual with an incredible amount of courage, strength, intelligence and drive. After polio, the last thing he needed was another challenge such as his lymphoma. Despite this, he was always ready for an aggressive approach to his illness which reflected the way, I believe, he treated life. Being involved in the care of such a remarkable man was truly an honor from my

perspective. In addition to all of his positive attributes, he always had time to show a twinkle in his eye, express a kind word and show off a smile that could light up a room. I truly looked forward and enjoyed all of my visits with him and will miss him.

I must say a word about your role in all of this. Your love and devotion for him was obvious from the start. You did everything you could to keep his life as normal as possible through the years of knowing you all. You were able to serve as both his medical advocate and loving family. This is a difficult road to walk to say the least, but you did so with an incredible amount of style and grace. You have markedly enhanced the quality of life of this extraordinary gentleman during the time that I have known you and should clearly harbor no guilt.

Again, while words are inadequate to express my feelings for both you and Ed, please accept my heartfelt condolences and please let me know if there is anything I can do for you at this time.

Sincerely,
Stephen C. Fox, M.D., FACP

LIVES TOUCHED BY ED

These adults wanted to share what Ed meant to them when they were children.

Joe Bernard

I was an impressionable 13 year old when I first met Ed. There was plenty of trouble to be found around the city and I could have gotten mixed up with a bad crowd, and probably still did. But Ed would have none of that. He'd see me riding my bike around on a Saturday afternoon and ask if I was going to be down at Coyne field for the weekly pickup baseball games he organized. If I said no, he'd ask what I was doing instead. If he didn't approve of what I was doing, he'd say something like "why do you want to do that and get yourself into trouble? Just get your butt over to the field tonight". I always seemed to find my way to the field, thanks to Ed. I learned a lot from Ed about being a good person, being a father, and being a friend. If at the end of my life I can become half the man that Ed was, I'll be a better man than most.

Jeffrey Benway

My memories of Ed begin with him taking me in as a young boy with all sisters and no father figure, a broken home, and a mom working three jobs to support us kids. We were impressionable to say the least, and as we all know, young boys who get no guidance usually end up dead on drugs or in prison early in life. Well, Mr. Ed Sill took the time every week to take a group of us little fresh-mouth

100-mile-an-hour brats to Coyne field to play sports together, thus teaching us how to build relationships with other kids, how to get over shyness, and how to be more prompt and on time for things.

He would not allow us to swear or be disrespectful, or we wouldn't be allowed to participate. This loving, giving man taught me soooooooo much! Even in the bitter cold this man, who suffered with his mobility, would get dressed, go outside in the snow (!!) and toss a football. Or he would referee our games of three-on-three football or just watch us play in the snow.

The entire neighborhood was "his kids"—good kids, troubled kids, bad kids ("untaught"—no kids are bad). Although I'm now a 48-year-old grown man, I am living proof that if this angel hadn't guided me when I was "vulnerable," I'm assuring you I'd most likely not even be alive today!!!

Want to talk about a pillar in the community? Anywhere he ever went, a hundred people would say "hi" to him! He loved everyone and was loved back just as much. If the world had more people like him in it, it would be a better place to live today!

After some time to think, I remember other things about Ed (LOL)—like his constant Green Bay wool hat, or maybe it was the Steelers but I'm thinking Green Bay. He attended Little League, Babe Ruth, girls' games, for every sport he was there for the kids. Coyne Field should be renamed "Edward Sill Memorial Park!"

Michael Jordan, Babe Ruth, Mickey Mantle, my hardworking mother—these are my heroes. My other hero was Mr. Ed Sill—a man who honestly wanted to improve life for everyone. He got no pay, no trophies, he just gave and gave. If there's a ballgame in heaven, Mr. Sill is either watching it, umpiring it, or most likely is the man who organized it!

If the letters "ED SILL" stand for something, it is "Every Day Saving Innocent Little Lives." What a man! To this day, when I drive down Green Street, I slow down, look at that house, and just reflect on the days of splendor I received there.

—Jeffrey Benway

Christopher S West

Ed had a huge impact on me and the neighborhood; I thought of him as a second dad, he was an inspiration to all. A man with a huge disability and he made it seem like it was nothing. It was almost like it didn't exist, it made him who he was, like my dad, and I don't remember either of them any other way.

I wouldn't have become who I am if it wasn't for the people in my life. I wouldn't change a thing. I remember those jar openers he put all over Kenny's car and how mad he was ("vote for stix") I will always laugh when I think of it. The impression he left on me is, live every day the best you can, and enjoy your kids—just as he was such a part of their lives.

—Christopher West

Rozell Family testimonial on behalf of Mark Rozell

For the Rozell family, who lived on Second Avenue in Rensselaer, NY from 1960 to 1978, Ed Sill was not just the "man down the street who walked with metal crutches," he was a surrogate father to our brother Mark and a friend to the rest of the family. Mark was a special needs child. We never knew his exact diagnosis but today believe he had Asperger's Syndrome. Mark died in 1980 from injuries sustained from an automobile accident.

Mark was a kind child, incapable of being mean or evil, yet he had very few friends his own age. Ed Sill was one of Mark's best friends growing up. Mark did not have a father in his life and Ed filled that void. Mark "chose" to love Ed and Ed "chose" to love Mark. There was no good reason why they should be friends, but they were.

Mark, with his special needs, was different. And, Ed, with his metal crutches, was also different. In being different they found that they were the same—kind, considerate, humorous, witty, and compassionate. Studies show that outside of genetics, those who we hang around with while growing up will have the most influence on the kind of person we will become. Mark was a great kid partially because of good genes, but also because of Ed Sill.

When Mark died, it was as if Ed lost one of his own children. And, for us, when Ed passed away, it was as if we lost a family member. Both are gone, but both will never be forgotten for the good deeds that they did and for the good memories that they have left behind.

—The Rozell Family

Larry Myers

Wow—so many stories and memories. My first memory of Ed "Sticks" Sill was when I was a Babe Ruth baseball player in Rensselaer. When I was 13 years old I was at the Boys Club in the city on a Saturday afternoon, and there was registration for Babe Ruth baseball that day so I signed up. I talked to Ed and Mrs. Foust and Mrs. Goca about the league. I was on the P.B.A. team and the coaches were Paul Benedetto, Kevin Perotte, and his brother I think, Michael Perotte.

I would hang around Coyne Field after the games and help put equipment away. Ed would always direct us to where things went in "The Shack" and would give me a ride home after all the work was done. Ed was very kind to a lot of kids in Rensselaer—there was always a group hanging around with Ed. After I was too old to play, Ed was instrumental in making me the scorekeeper and announcer at Coyne field for Babe Ruth and also the Rensselaer Night Softball League.

I would also attend the league meetings at the Broadway firehouse; Ed was president of the league.

After the baseball schedule was over, the boys would go fishing and swimming with Ed, every other Saturday. He took the girls on the alternate weekends. For three bucks we would get into the "Blue Boat," or as Ed called it his "Chevy Impala." It had Liquid Nails sealant around all the window trim to keep the leaks at bay. We would go to Kinderhook Lake and rent a boat or two and fish for a couple of hours. We would bring a lunch and row to an island and eat lunch. Ed always brought a big thermos jug of Kool-Aid. We would eat lunch and then go fishing some more. I know his wife, Sandie wasn't too happy when we got back and would clean the fish in the back yard, but we always cleaned up our mess. If our fishing day was rained out we would hang out with Ed anyway, helping him in his workshop in the cellar on Green Street.

Ed took a bunch of us on driving lessons numerous times, at the high school parking lot on Broadway, driving around the parking lot with the parking lines and the road around the front of the school. I went for walks with Ed around the city. Even though Ed had polio and walked with crutches, he never let his disability prevent him from going on his walks. We would look on the ground for "treasure"—old bolts and things; Ed had jars full of these things at home, we would pick up every nail or screw we saw, because as Ed said, "This, my boy, could damage a tire and we don't want that."

When Ed was campaigning for Alderman for his Ward, he "employed" some of the kids to help him "get the word out." We would bring newsletters and campaign stuff to all of the houses in Ed's Ward, things like rubber discs for jar openers, pencils, small pads of paper, and little gift bags.

When I read the obit in the Times Union I was really heartbroken. I had so many great memories of Ed. There are so many other stories, like when the rope line for home runs was up at Coyne field. I remember some of the people—Charlie Romano, Kevin Perotte, Don Brady, Ruth Foust, June Goca, June Glass, and Hooper Van Vorst. I remember the charity softball game against FLY-92. There are a lot more stories to tell...

—Larry Myers

Frank Faccioli

Wow, when I was asked to write something that I remembered the most about Mr. Sill, there were so many things that came to mind, like my first fishing experience or the first time I played baseball and so many other things. Ed was for sure like a father to me, and being the youngest on the street at that time I needed that.

But there was one time in particular—my favorite story. We used to take these walks through the city of Rensselaer in upstate New York. I would somehow get conned into taking this walk with him. One day it was just him and me. I remember when I look back at it now, he listen when I talked. We would talk about school and sports and stuff, but he knew that music was my love. He would tell me, "Frankie, if that's what you want to do than that's what you do but don't be good at it, be great at it."

I remember us walking, picking up bottles along the way, and anyone who has taken this walk with him knows what that means. At the end of the walk we would dispose of them in a very cool way. Well as a kid, it's cool. We would smash them against a wall that was kind of like a waterfall (and to not get in trouble for it, that was the cool part). He was very into keeping the streets clean of litter and things like that.

I watched him as a man I could trust; his love for his family and his wife were incredible to say the least. As a man today, I find myself doing things that he did with my family, it was family first and he was there for all of them. When thinking of all the moments I had with this family, it was you Mr. Sill, who made me want to have more in life than just being another kid from the streets. Thank you for putting up with me. I miss you and love you. God above has a great man with him.

—Frank Faccioli (one of kids in the neighborhood

that was touched by him)

OTHER PEOPLE'S REMEMBRANCES

Here are some of the comments that people from work had sent us and comments put on cards at the two services we had for him—one in Pennsylvania, where all of his co-workers were and one in Rensselaer, where we spent most of our lives.

"I remember most Ed's optimism and his delight in telling stories about his friends and family. He enjoyed his time, as a treasured gift, which he opened every day and shared with those around him. Each of us could benefit with Ed's approach to life as our lives touch others at home and at work."
—John Gray

"While my wife, Maria, was going through her own difficulties with terminal cancer, I related the story of the struggles Ed was having and had been going through over many years in his efforts to enjoy just one more day of life…and another, then another. Through that example of his courage, he gave strength and courage to others facing difficulties in their own daily struggles with illness, a shining example indeed to a person who never previously had the privilege of meeting him. I remember him fondly for being that example and will always be grateful for his gift of courage and inspiration to others. Thanks, Ed."

—Rafael & Maria Rosario

"There are many wonderful words that could be used to describe Ed. But chief among them is "inspiration". I worked closely with Ed during his last two years here at Sanofi and to me that was a great benefit. He was always encouraging, was always engaging, and could brighten anyone's day. He had a quality that made it easy for me to come to work—not just a day on the job, but a day with Ed! This I will always miss because they've "broken the mold". He loved people and understood what mattered to them; what others felt was important. What did he bring to the office every day? Some wisdom? A piece of advice? A kind word? Charm? Light humor and great moments of hilarity to break the monotony? Yes, each day he carried all these things with him and much more—the page is too short to list them all. He touched countless lives and made them better. He touched my life and made it better."

—Dusty

Ed was a true inspiration to me for many, many years. There was a time when I was struggling through a very bad divorce. I would come to work upset and see Ed in the hall. I would say, "Hi Ed, how are you?" His answer was always "FANTASTIC!" If Ed could be fantastic, then the least I could do was to see that my problems, no matter how bad they were, would pass and I could straighten up my own attitude and put a smile on my face. He was a kind, sweet, brave, funny, wonderful man and I missed him when he left Sanofi and will continue to miss him. I offer my deepest condolences and prayers to all his family."

—Anonymous

"I met Ed for the first time in 1993 after he was returning to work from a cancer treatment. I was impressed with Ed's great outgoing personality. The next day I happened to see Ed at a local store and found out he lived only a mile from me. I asked him if he would like to ride to work with me and Ed thought that would be great. Our friendship would grow quickly and soon spread between our families. Our family ties would become even closer with the marriage of his daughter and my nephew. The past twelve years passed much too soon but will always hold many great memories of the many things we have done over the years. We had so many great times at work and at home, I can't even begin to write them down. I am sure we will remain close throughout the years."

—Barry

Barry was diagnosed with cancer and passed away the year after Ed passed. The car pool buddies are together again.

"The times we had at Lake St. Catherine, swimming, playing, horseshoes and picnics. You were a courageous brother-in-law. We'll miss you! Love,"

—Linda & family

"A man who took me under his wing and gave me the experience of what a true father is. A family taking care of me like one of their own. Who else could have taught me how to gut a fish? Or how to drive? These are only the tip of the iceberg of what I learned and felt from a most precious man. I will be lost in thoughts of you always Dad!!!"

—Lisa

"Ed, I have never met a man with as big a heart and such a fire for life. You will be sorely missed. I always looked forward to the talks we had and football season. Thanks for all that you have done for me. Getting me started when we first moved to the neighborhood with firewood that a friend of yours had. I will always remember you as my neighbor but most of all a good friend. My mother is waiting to say hello to you. Love you always,"

—The Lewars Family

"Always thinking of others and thinking of himself last. Ed brought happiness and laughter to everyone he met. Love, compassion, honor and trust are just a few qualities of Ed. Ed knows how to go with the flow and always finds the positive. Laughter, humor, and joking, Ed always knew how to keep life lighthearted. I will always remember Ed as my best friend."

—Robert D. Tocher

"All the happy camp days at Lake St. Catherine. My house and pool with all the family gatherings. Your positive attitude no matter how ill you felt. All the family nicknames and your happy smile. Your kids' love for you. Sandie's love for you. Thank you for all the smiles. Rest in peace—I know you're already playing golf with Bill. Much love,"

—Jane

"It always brightened my day to see you outside. You would always greet me and you were so kind and generous to everyone. No matter how you were doing you always kept a smile on. I'm going to miss seeing you on my walks in the summer outside. You made the sunny days even brighter. The street won't be the same without you. Love,"

—Lindsay

"Moving to Reading in October, 2002, thinking it was your typical neighborhood, you were the first person who greeted us and I quickly questioned typical. Ed, we have had so many good times together I thought of you as a mentor. There are only two things I will ever regret having known you,... letting you supervise me while I was painting my house and today. I love and will miss you always,"

—Ryan, Beth, Reagan Ginsberg

When Ed passed away, Beth made up Green and Yellow Bows and went around the neighborhood to ask neighbors if they would put one on their mailbox in memory of Ed. So when we came home one day, the whole block had these Green Bay Packer bows on their mailbox posts and I just cried. What a loving memory, he would have loved to see that.

"Of course, I remember the teasing and name calling. Who could forget the "Styrofoam mosaic walls" in the basement. However, the most important thing that I remember is how Ed would respond with "Terrific!" when you asked him how he was doing, no matter what current health struggle he was going through. That made all the difference. Thank you for this lesson, Ed."

—Donna

Sandie

This is a poem that I saved from a card I gave to him many years ago, I felt it described him as a special husband. Have no idea who the author is. Here is how it went:

Edward & Sandra Sill

This Is a Husband

A husband is that special man
You would write a book about.
The one you love to be with
And couldn't do without.

A husband is a gentle look,
A hand within your own,
He always makes you proud
To feel that you are his alone.

A husband understands your moods
And laughs at things you say;
He sees you when you're at your worst
And loves you anyway.

A husband is the one you kiss
And make up with again
When there's a little difference
Of opinion now and then.

He is that special man who shares
All that you're dreaming of,
And gives a magic meaning
To the wonder that is love.

I felt Ed was a special person when meeting him. He had such a great attitude about things and was willing to try most things even though he was physically challenged. After that first kiss, I was hooked. He had a great kindness in his heart for everyone's battles, was a lot of fun to be with and had interesting stories. He definitely wasn't perfect, as there was also this stubborn streak that sometimes would cause an argument... but if you could prove to him the other way was right, he would concede. Life wasn't always good, we had a couple of separations, but usually not for long. We seemed to be able to talk about our differences and work things out. He was a great lover, confidante, husband, and a great father. I miss his presence, his hugs and kisses, but feel that he is now in a better place, as seeing him suffer for those last few years was very hard for all of us to watch. I'm sure that the Lord has him as the greeter at the Golden Gates... ha, ha, ha... as he loved talking to everyone. Hoping what I have written is some of the things Ed wanted to share with all of you. Surely there is a lot left out, but hopefully some of you who knew him can fill in the blanks.

My children and I thank all of our family, neighbors and friends for all their assistance and love with helping Ed and I through some of these tough times and for all the fun times we enjoyed with you. Ed and I had talked a lot about special times and memories before he passed and how thankful we are for the wonderful life and friends that came in and out of our lives. The fun we had bringing up our children and, of course, the trials and blessings they have given us. He loved his family so much and did not want to leave us, but knew that his body wasn't cooperating with his mind. He will always be in our hearts no matter how much time goes by.

Special thanks to Ed's sisters Patty and Rena for the some of the pictures that they contributed. Thanks to my children for all of their input, support, and guidance with this book. Also, to our grandchildren, friends and all of the wonderful people that contributed their thoughts about Ed. I especially want to thank Dick Conklin, who went to high school with Ed (Guilderland Central HS), for his assistance in editing and helping me put this book together, also for finding some old newspaper articles about Ed. THANK YOU SOOOO MUCH.

"I remember Ed in high school. He was a great guy and easy to talk to, with a great sense of humor. We lived only a couple of miles apart, just off Western Avenue. Ed and I met again at a high school reunion many years later. I had written some books and Ed asked me if I could help him with a book he wanted to write (this one). Unfortunately, Ed died before he could finish it, but Sandie picked up where he left off and it has been a great privilege to work with her to complete this project. I knew most of the high school buddies that Ed talked about in this book and unfortunately I have had to write obituaries for many of them on our Web site, keysy.com/gchs59."

—Dick Conklin, GCHS Class of 1959, Ponce Inlet, Florida

Bruce Gauvin

Bruce is a friend who worked with Ed at Sterling Winthrop and was also one of the players on the various sports teams. This is what he recalls about Ed:

> When I think about Ed, "Unflappable" comes immediately to mind. He was my inspiration. He was the inspiration for many.
>
> Knowing Ed for several decades was my blessing. On the wall over my desk at work I had a picture of Ed—a simple picture of a great man that illustrated who and what he was. Here was Big Ed in a bathing suit, sitting in shallow water at a lake shoreline. Several sunfish were swimming around and went right up to him to take bread crumbs out of his hand. Knowing how I loved to fish, he would say, "This is how you catch them, Bruce." All the Lord's creations adored him... or maybe it was that Green Bay Packers Cheese Head hat he wore.
>
> If ever there was a Readers Digest "Most Unforgettable Character," it was Ed.
>
> This was the picture I'd look at or recall when confronted by one of the many lifetime stresses that came

along. It was my solace. It was also the story I told to others who were going through stress or similar health-related battles. Telling it not only lighted up my eyes, it was a great enjoyment to watch others begin smiling with hope.

Rena

Ed's sister Rena provided photographs and comments which appear at the end of this chapter.

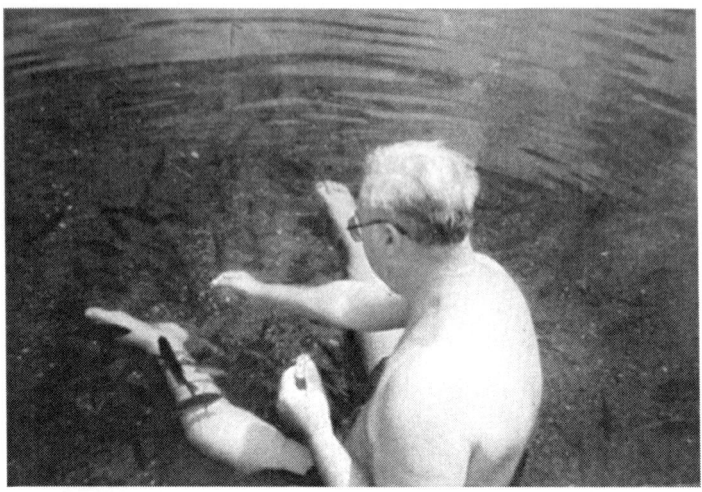

Ed feeding sunfish. Bruce Gauvin recalls this photo fondly.

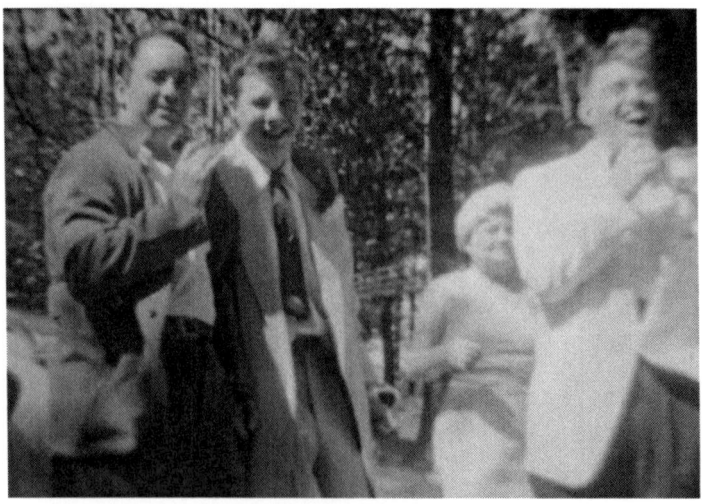

Ed shortly after returning home from the hospital. He is holding onto the handle of his Canadian crutches. This photo and the ones on pages 169–170 were provided by Ed's sister, Rena.

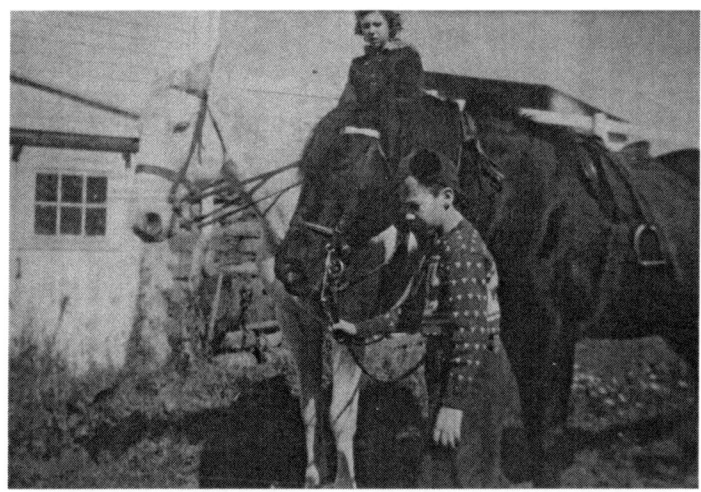

This photo with horses was taken when Ed was 10 or 12 years old.

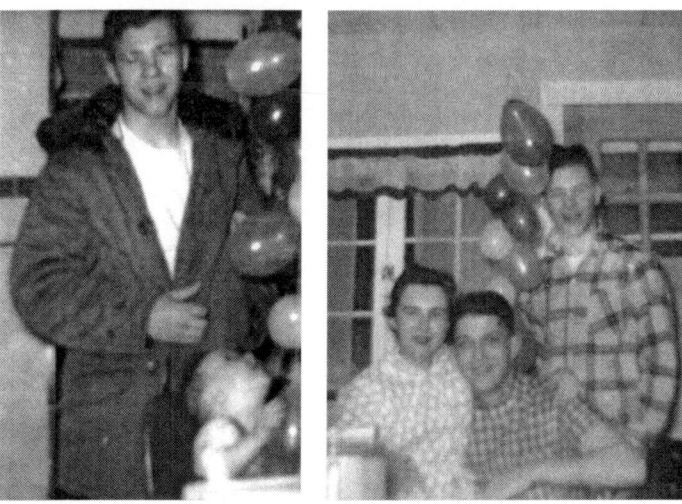

These Church Road photos were taken just before he came down with polio. Rena said she will never forget the horror of that diagnosis for him and the family. *Right:* Rena and her husband Jerry with Ed.

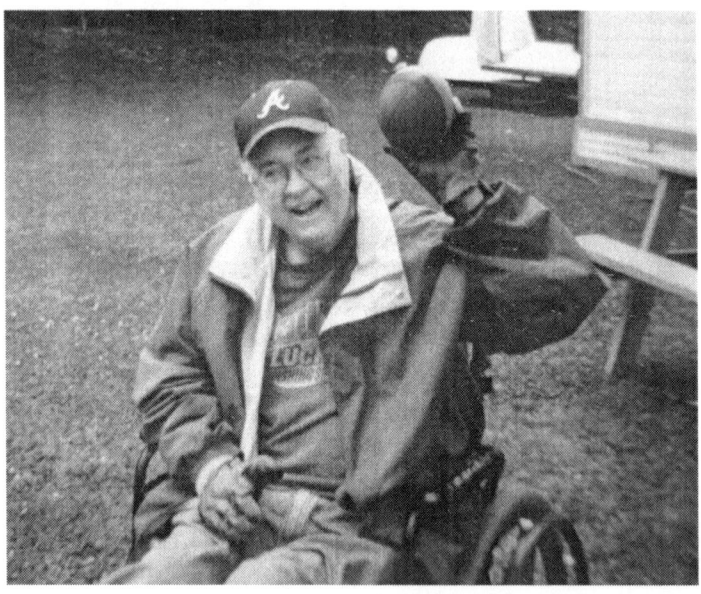

Ed at Lake St. Catherine several years before he passed. He wore gloves and coats most of the time because he was always cold, even in the summertime.

CPSIA information can be obtained at www.ICGtesting.com
Printed in the USA
BVOW031836190812

298106BV00001BA/2/P